NATIONAL ACADEMIES

Sciences
Engineering
Medicine

NATIONAL
ACADEMIES
PRESS
Washington, DC

Assessing Intake of Food and Dietary Supplements in Older Adults

T0315518

Emily A. Callahan and Hoda Soltani,
Rapporteurs

Food and Nutrition Board

Health and Medicine Division

Proceedings of a Workshop Series

NATIONAL ACADEMIES PRESS 500 Fifth Street, NW, Washington, DC 20001

This activity was supported by a contract between the National Academy of Sciences and the National Institutes of Health's Office of Dietary Supplements (contract no. HHSN263201800029I). Any opinions, findings, conclusions, or recommendations expressed in this publication do not necessarily reflect the views of any organization or agency that provided support for the project.

International Standard Book Number-13: 978-0-309-69561-9
International Standard Book Number-10: 0-309-69561-9
Digital Object Identifier: https://doi.org/10.17226/26771

This publication is available from the National Academies Press, 500 Fifth Street, NW, Keck 360, Washington, DC 20001; (800) 624-6242 or (202) 334-3313; http://www.nap.edu.

Suggested citation: National Academies of Sciences, Engineering, and Medicine. 2023. *Assessing intake of food and dietary supplements in older adults: Proceedings of a workshop series*. Washington, DC: The National Academies Press. https://doi.org/10.17226/26771.

The **National Academy of Sciences** was established in 1863 by an Act of Congress, signed by President Lincoln, as a private, nongovernmental institution to advise the nation on issues related to science and technology. Members are elected by their peers for outstanding contributions to research. Marcia McNutt is president.

The **National Academy of Engineering** was established in 1964 under the charter of the National Academy of Sciences to bring the practices of engineering to advising the nation. Members are elected by their peers for extraordinary contributions to engineering. John L. Anderson is president.

The **National Academy of Medicine** (formerly the Institute of Medicine) was established in 1970 under the charter of the National Academy of Sciences to advise the nation on medical and health issues. Members are elected by their peers for distinguished contributions to medicine and health. Victor J. Dzau is president.

The three Academies work together as the **National Academies of Sciences, Engineering, and Medicine** to provide independent, objective analysis and advice to the nation and conduct other activities to solve complex problems and inform public policy decisions. The National Academies also encourage education and research, recognize outstanding contributions to knowledge, and increase public understanding in matters of science, engineering, and medicine.

Learn more about the National Academies of Sciences, Engineering, and Medicine at **www.nationalacademies.org**.

Consensus Study Reports published by the National Academies of Sciences, Engineering, and Medicine document the evidence-based consensus on the study's statement of task by an authoring committee of experts. Reports typically include findings, conclusions, and recommendations based on information gathered by the committee and the committee's deliberations. Each report has been subjected to a rigorous and independent peer-review process and it represents the position of the National Academies on the statement of task.

Proceedings published by the National Academies of Sciences, Engineering, and Medicine chronicle the presentations and discussions at a workshop, symposium, or other event convened by the National Academies. The statements and opinions contained in proceedings are those of the participants and are not endorsed by other participants, the planning committee, or the National Academies.

Rapid Expert Consultations published by the National Academies of Sciences, Engineering, and Medicine are authored by subject-matter experts on narrowly focused topics that can be supported by a body of evidence. The discussions contained in rapid expert consultations are considered those of the authors and do not contain policy recommendations. Rapid expert consultations are reviewed by the institution before release.

For information about other products and activities of the National Academies, please visit www.nationalacademies.org/about/whatwedo.

PLANNING COMMITTEE ON ASSESSING INTAKE OF FOOD AND DIETARY SUPPLEMENTS IN OLDER ADULTS[1]

CAROL J. BOUSHEY (*Chair*), Associate Research Professor, Epidemiology Program, University of Hawai'i Cancer Center

REGAN L. BAILEY, Associate Institute Director, Institute for Advancing Health through Agriculture, and Professor of Nutrition, Texas A&M University

CLARE CORISH, Professor of Clinical Nutrition & Dietetics and Program Director, Masters in Clinical Nutrition & Dietetics, School of Public Health, Physiotherapy and Sports Science, University College Dublin

DIANE MITCHELL, Associate Research Professor and Director of the Diet Assessment Center in the Department of Nutritional Sciences, Pennsylvania State University

ROSE ANN DiMARIA-GHALILI, Senior Associate Dean for Research and Professor of Nursing, College of Nursing and Health Professions, Drexel University

ELBERT HUANG, Professor of Medicine and Public Health Sciences and Director, Center for Chronic Disease Research and Policy, University of Chicago

GORDON L. JENSEN, Senior Associate Dean for Research and Professor of Medicine and Nutrition, Emeritus, Larner College of Medicine, University of Vermont

HEATHER KELLER, Schlegel Research Chair in Nutrition & Aging, Schlegel-University of Waterloo Research Institute for Aging, and Professor, Department of Kinesiology and Health Sciences, University of Waterloo

Health and Medicine Division Staff

HODA SOLTANI, Senior Program Officer
NICOLE CUNNINGHAM, Research Associate
ANN L. YAKTINE, Director, Food and Nutrition Board

---

[1]The National Academies of Sciences, Engineering, and Medicine's planning committees are solely responsible for organizing the workshop, identifying topics, and choosing speakers. The responsibility for the published Proceedings of a Workshop rests with the workshop rapporteurs and the institution.

Reviewers

This Proceedings of a Workshop Series was reviewed in draft form by individuals chosen for their diverse perspectives and technical expertise. The purpose of this independent review is to provide candid and critical comments that will assist the National Academies of Sciences, Engineering, and Medicine in making each published proceedings as sound as possible and to ensure that it meets the institutional standards for quality, objectivity, evidence, and responsiveness to the charge. The review comments and draft manuscript remain confidential to protect the integrity of the process. We thank the following individuals for their review of this proceedings:

ROSE ANN DiMARIA-GHALILI, Senior Associate Dean for Research and Professor of Nursing, College of Nursing and Health Professions, Drexel University

MARIE KAINOA FIALKOWSKI REVILLA, Associate Professor in Human Nutrition, University of Hawai'i at Mānoa

Although the reviewers listed above provided many constructive comments and suggestions, they were not asked to endorse the content of the proceedings, nor did they see the final draft before its release. The review of this proceedings was overseen by **CHERYL ANDERSON**, Herbert Wertheim School of Public Health, University of California, San Diego. She was responsible for making certain that an independent examination of this proceedings was carried out in accordance with standards of the National Academies and that all review comments were carefully considered. Responsibility for the final content rests entirely with the rapporteurs and the National Academies. We also thank staff member Lida Beninson for reading and providing helpful comments on this manuscript.

Contents

Boxes and Figures

1

Introduction

Dietary assessment in older adults presents many unique problems due to the diversity of health states and capabilities that span the population group. Additional complications are created by variations in intakes due to illnesses, medications affecting appetite, altered sensory modalities and cognition, and the variety of living arrangements. Although a good deal is known about dietary intakes, body composition, and nutritional status among the "young old" (arbitrarily defined as 65–74), who tend to be relatively free of chronic degenerative diseases and conditions, very little is known about those 75+ and particularly the very old (85 and older). These individuals are often affected by multiple morbidities, polypharmacy, functional deficits, and alterations in body composition that all increase with age, and all of these have potent impacts on nutritional status and complicate dietary assessment. Many of the common medications older adults take regularly affect nutritional status, so information on medications must also be taken into account in assessments.

Many individuals aged 80 years and older are generally able to perform well in dietary studies; however, some may report food habits from earlier in life. Identifying those older adults who may not able to respond correctly to standard intake assessment approaches, such as 24-hour recalls or food frequency questionnaires (FFQs), will require adapted techniques, such as observation of intakes and outputs in hospitalized patients and other food records. Such challenges to accurate dietary assessment warrant exploration of better methodologies to support both basic and translational research on older adults.

A virtual workshop series titled Assessing Intake of Food and Dietary Supplements in Older Adults was convened in spring 2022 by the Food and Nutrition Board, Health and Medicine Division, National Academies of Sciences, Engineering, and Medicine. The series was planned by a committee[1] of experts and included four virtual workshops (held April 8, April 22, April 29, and May 6) intended to provide guidance to researchers and clinicians. The workshops aimed to outline considerations relating to different methods of assessing intakes of food and dietary supplements in older adults, with special emphasis on those 75 and older. The broad topics covered included current status of dietary and nutrition assessment of older adults and advances and key issues in this topic; nutritional screening of older adults; and nutritional practices, challenges, and policies that affect older adults. The workshop's statement of task is in Box 1-1.[2]

ORGANIZATION OF THIS PROCEEDINGS

This proceedings follows the order of the four workshop agendas (Appendix A), chronicling each workshop in its own chapter. Chapter 2 explores demographic trends and the current state of research on nutritional assessment in aging populations (workshop 1); Chapter 3 examines recent studies and developments in creating and applying dietary assessment tools for aging populations (workshop 2); Chapter 4 reviews recent research on screening for undernutrition in aging populations (workshop 3); and Chapter 5 explores the broader landscape and policies surrounding the nutritional assessment of older adults (workshop 4). Appendix B is a list of acronyms used in this proceedings, and Appendix C provides biographical sketches of each workshop's speakers and planning committee members.

---

[1] The planning committee's role was limited to planning the workshop, and the Proceedings of a Workshop has been prepared by the workshop rapporteurs as a factual summary of what occurred at the workshop. Statements, recommendations, and opinions expressed are those of individual presenters and participants, and are not necessarily endorsed or verified by the National Academies of Sciences, Engineering, and Medicine, and they should not be construed as reflecting any group consensus.

[2] The workshop agenda, presentations, and other materials are available at https://www.nationalacademies.org/our-work/assessing-intake-of-food-and-dietary-supplements-in-older-adults-a-workshop-series.

BOX 1-1
Workshop Statement of Task

A planning committee of the National Academies of Sciences, Engineering, and Medicine will plan a series of three to four public virtual workshops that explore the evidence on methods for best practices in assessing dietary intakes and instituting more harmonization and standardization in applying those methods to assess dietary intakes in older adults, with special emphasis on those 75 years of age and older. The workshops will feature invited presentations and discussions focused on providing guidance to researchers and clinicians. Specific issues to be considered include

1. Methods to improve assessment of oral intake from all sources (food, beverages, drugs, supplements) in older adults, with an emphasis on subgroups (i.e., by chronological age [old, oldest old], biological age [healthy and frail], functional status, literacy level, settings [i.e., community-living, assisted-living, and long-term chronic care facilities, nursing homes, hospitals], program participation [i.e., home-delivered meal programs, Commodity Supplemental Food Program, Supplemental Nutrition Assistance Program, the Emergency Food Assistance Program]);
2. Summaries of what is known and not known (gaps in knowledge) about total dietary intakes in older adults, especially those identifying gaps in dietary assessment tools used and possible remedies for them, and the special challenges in older adult populations, which are relevant to the Dietary Guidelines 2025–2030 which will focus on older adults; and
3. Exploration of best practices and guidelines for total dietary assessment for surveillance and clinical care (i.e., oral intake from foods, beverages, dietary supplements, and medications) in older adult groups and subgroups residing in various settings.

The planning committee will organize the workshop, select and invite speakers and discussants, and moderate the discussions. Workshop proceedings of the presentations and discussions will be prepared by a designated rapporteur in accordance with institutional guidelines.

2

Foundations and Current Status of Dietary and Nutrition Assessment of Older Adults

---

BOX 2-1
HIGHLIGHTS[a]

- The rapid aging of populations around the globe—individuals aged 65 and older comprise 25–30 percent of the population in many countries—and the increase in life expectancy at age 65 in many countries point to the timeliness and importance of discussing the role of diet in healthy aging. (Keller)
- According to estimates of malnutrition in community-dwelling older adults at a national level, which were produced via secondary analysis of the National Health and Aging Trends Study longitudinal cohort, 68 percent have normal nutrition status, 26 percent are at risk for malnutrition, and about 6 percent are malnourished. (DiMaria-Ghalili)
- The Longitudinal Aging Study Amsterdam recorded a nearly 70 percent response rate when participants were invited to undergo dietary assessment by completing a food frequency questionnaire (FFQ). Validation studies indicated that the FFQ validity was as good in older adults as in younger adults and similar to that of FFQs for older adults from other countries. (Visser)
- Results of longitudinal studies consistently suggest that lower adherence to healthy dietary patterns is associated with consequences among older adults, such as reduced mobility, accelerated decline in cognitive function, and accelerated development of frailty. Metabolite presence and levels can serve as an objective measure of dietary quality. (Ferrucci)
- The nutritionDay initiative is a 1-day, cross-sectional audit on nutrition care held annually in hospitals and nursing homes. It collects data on residents' and patients' food intakes, which are included in a large database that is avail-

---

able for analysis, but energy and nutrient intake information are not collected. (Volkert)

- A majority of older adults routinely use at least one dietary supplement. Whereas many older adults were found to be at risk of inadequate intake, based on food and beverage intake alone, for nutrients such as calcium, magnesium, zinc, folate, vitamin B6, vitamin B12, vitamin C, and vitamin D, including dietary supplements considerably reduces the proportion of those at risk for those nutrients. (Jun)

---

[a] This list is the rapporteurs' summary of points made by the individual speakers identified, and the statements have not been endorsed or verified by the National Academies of Sciences, Engineering, and Medicine. They are not intended to reflect a consensus among workshop participants.

The first workshop, held April 8, 2022, featured an introductory session about global demographic changes, five presentations that described datasets for dietary assessment of older adults, and a panel discussion with the workshop speakers. The datasets and surveys discussed included nutritionDay,[1] the Baltimore Longitudinal Study on Aging and InChianti Study, National Health and Nutrition Examination Survey (NHANES), National Health and Aging Trends Study (NHATS), and Longitudinal Aging Study Amsterdam (LASA).

INTRODUCTION: CHANGING DEMOGRAPHICS

Heather Keller, University of Waterloo (UW) and Schlegel-UW Research Institute for Aging, presented a brief overview of global demographic trends to illustrate the timeliness and importance of discussing the role of diet in healthy aging. She shared maps from the United Nations (UN) Population Division that illustrate the rapid aging of the world's population. The first map distinguished countries based on the percentage of their population aged 65 and older (Figure 2-1). In 1950, that was only 5–10 percent in almost all countries, whereas nearly 70 years later, it comprises more than 10 percent and up to 25–30 percent in many countries.

In addition to the rapid aging of populations worldwide, Keller continued, an increase in life expectancy at age 65 has occurred in many countries, and the gap between countries on this metric has narrowed overall (UN DESA Population Division, 2019). The UN projections of life expectancy at birth for individuals born between 2025 and 2030 indicate that much

---

[1] www.nutritionday.org (accessed September 14, 2022).

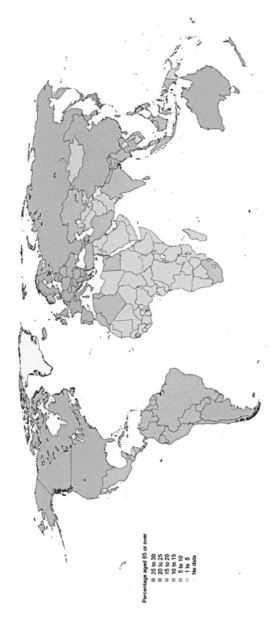

FIGURE 2-1 Percentage of populations aged 65 and older in countries worldwide.
SOURCE: Presented by Heather Keller on April 8, 2022 (UN DESA Population Division, 2019).

of the world will be expected to live beyond 70, and a sizable proportion will be expected to live beyond 80 (UN DESA Population Division, 2019). Keller underscored the importance of considering the impact of these shifts on population health, and she highlighted the role of diet in healthy aging. According to a study that put forth nine habits for longevity (Buettner and Skemp, 2016), two of them are directly related to diet—eat plants and stop eating when 80 percent full.

Keller relayed that the World Health Organization (WHO) has recognized demographic changes and designated 2021–2030 as a "decade of healthy aging." In its baseline report on healthy aging, WHO described it as a "process of developing and maintaining functional ability that enables well-being in older age" (WHO, 2021), which Keller said essentially equates functional ability with not being frail. Diet is closely connected with frailty, a condition that often overlaps with sarcopenia and malnutrition. Frailty can result from a variety of contributing factors, and diet probably plays a role (WHO, 2021).

NUTRITIONDAY

Dorothee Volkert, Friedrich-Alexander-University of Erlangen-Nürnberg, discussed nutritionDay, a worldwide, 1-day cross-sectional audit on nutrition care held annually in hospitals and nursing homes. NutritionDay is an awareness initiative that was adopted to improve knowledge about disease-related malnutrition and nutrition care and improve patient safety by monitoring quality of nutrition care globally. Its vision is to achieve standardized nutritional assessment in all institutions and a discussion of malnutrition as a public health concern at the political level. Institutions are invited to participate for free, and standardized questionnaires are available for local nursing staff to collect data and enter them in a joined online database.

Volkert focused on the nursing home setting for the nutritionDay initiative, explaining that the focus is on older adult residents, in contrast to the hospital settings, where patients of all ages can participate. She shared examples of nursing home questionnaires—one for collecting information about the institution, including characteristics such as unit size and nutritional routines; another for collecting information about individual residents; and a third for 6-month follow-up data collection, which tracks mortality, hospital admissions, and falls. Only three questions on the resident questionnaire are concerned with nutrition and food intake, and they ask about intake during a given day, the past week, and the past 3 months.

She highlighted the large size of the nutritionDay database as a strength and the absence of energy and nutrient intake information as a limitation. Between 2007 (the year the initiative commenced) and 2015, that more than 30,000 residents from 20 countries were represented in the nursing home database, with an additional 10,000 residents from 17 countries participating from 2016 to 2020 (when a shorter version of the question-naires was in use). The initiative's database is available for analysis with a signed data use agreement and accepted research proposal submitted to the nutritionDay office. Volkert noted that data analysis may be performed by the nutritionDay office in Vienna or by researchers themselves. Several publications using the dataset are available, such as a descriptive analysis of indicators for reduced food intake (Schindler et al., 2016); research on prevalence and associated factors for low food intake in hospital patients from different medical specialties (Bohne et al., 2022); and an annual report highlighting that around one-third of nursing home residents ate half or less of the lunch meal on the annual assessment (Tarantino et al., 2022).

Volkert added a few comments about dietary assessment in institutions serving older adults. Such settings typically contain physically and/or men-tally impaired populations, which makes self-assessment of dietary intake via recall or records infeasible. On a positive note, the meal plan and menus are well known, with mostly standardized portions. Volkert suggested that nursing home staff perform dietary assessment using either plate diagrams to estimate the proportion of a meal or specific food items consumed, esti-mated food records, or weighed records—which are the gold standard but also the most laborious.

BALTIMORE LONGITUDINAL STUDY ON AGING AND INCHIANTI STUDY

Luigi Ferrucci, National Institute on Aging at the National Institutes of Health (NIH), shared data from the Baltimore Longitudinal Study on Aging (BLSA) and Invecchiare in Chianti ("aging in the Chianti area" [InChianti]) study. Ferrucci believed that nutrition is "the culprit of how we age"—aging and health are surely affected by food consumed throughout the lifetime.

Ferrucci described the dietary assessment component of the BLSA. This cohort study collected 3–7-day dietary records among a relatively healthy population between 1984 and 1992 and again between 1994 and 2003. The time and labor intensiveness of this practice led to its replacement with food frequency questionnaires (FFQs) in 2003, which is completed by the respondent or administered by an interviewer via phone or in person. BLSA examines respondents' adherence to three dietary patterns (and diet quality) that have been associated with positive health outcomes: Mediterranean, Mediterranean-DASH Intervention for Neurodegenerative Delay (MIND), and Alternate Healthy Eating Index (AHEI).

Ferrucci shared data on the percentage of BLSA participants with "high adherence" (i.e., top tertile based on a score that considers consumption frequency of various food groups and key nutrients) to one of these three dietary patterns (Figure 2-2). He pointed out a substantial age effect that is

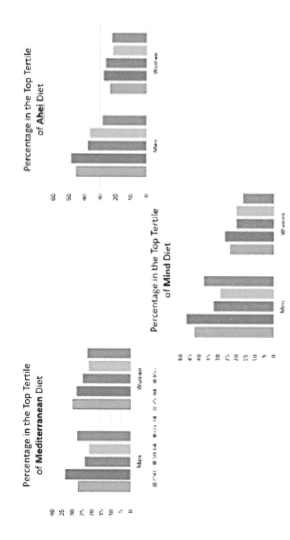

FIGURE 2-2 Percentage of Baltimore Longitudinal Study of Aging participants with high adherence (top tertile of adherence score) to healthy diets by age and sex.
SOURCE: Presented by Luigi Ferrucci on April 8, 2022.

seemingly sex dependent—women have an increasingly lower likelihood of high adherence to Mediterranean or MIND diets as age increases.

Ferrucci shared data on the relationships between varying levels of adherence to a Mediterranean-style diet and the health outcomes of mobility decline and frailty. In one cross-sectional analysis, all three tertiles of adherence (high, medium, and low) to the diet at baseline were nearly identical in terms of score for a key metric of mobility decline; but, over time, participants with low adherence showed a significant reduction in mobility compared to those with high adherence (Milaneschi et al., 2011). Another cross-sectional analysis demonstrated that higher adherence is inversely associated with developing frailty in community-dwelling older men and women (Talegawkar et al., 2012).

Ferrucci indicated that longitudinal data provide consistent results, which he illustrated with findings from a cohort study that observed accelerated frailty among participants with baseline frailty index (FI) measures below the median and low adherence to the Mediterranean diet during a 10-year follow-up period (Figure 2-3).

Another longitudinal study examined adherence to a Mediterranean diet and cognitive decline among participants in the InChianti study. During a follow-up period of nearly 20 years, Ferrucci reported that an accelerated decline in cognitive function was observed among participants who had low

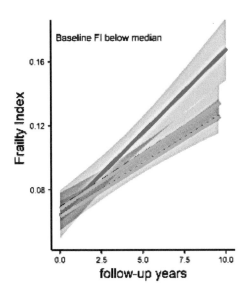

FIGURE 2-3 Association of adherence to the Mediterranean-style diet with lower frailty index (FI) in older adults.
SOURCE: Presented by Luigi Ferrucci on April 8, 2022 (Tanaka et al., 2021).

adherence (Tanaka et al., 2018). This effect seemed to be mostly attributable to intakes of vegetables, fish, legumes, and fruit and nuts.

Ferrucci also mentioned data on the relationship between varying levels of adherence to a MIND intervention diet and physical function and grip strength in older adults. He shared evidence of an accelerated decline in physical health among participants in the lowest tertile of adherence (Talegawkar et al., 2022).

According to Ferrucci, reporting bias is a challenge of dietary assessment. To address this, his group is working to evaluate dietary intake using blood and urine biomarkers. Ferrucci shared a study that found a strong correlation between total urinary polyphenol and mortality but a null effect between the two when total dietary polyphenol was calculated on a participant-reported questionnaire (Zamora-Ros et al., 2013). He suggested that the best approach is probably a combination of self-reported and objective dietary assessment tools.

Ferrucci moved on to potential mechanisms by which the different diets affect health outcomes. One effect is certainly epigenetic, given evidence indicating that consuming fish, fruits, and vegetables; moderating alcohol intake; high socioeconomic status and level of education; and regular physical activity were associated with a "slower epigenetic clock" (a slower progression of aging; Quach et al., 2017). In contrast, central obesity, high triglyceride and low HDL cholesterol values, high systolic blood pressure, presence of inflammatory markers, dysregulated insulin function/elevated glucose levels, and meat consumption were associated with faster epigenetic aging.

Another mechanism by which diet affects health is the metabolites that are produced as a result of dietary intakes, Ferrucci continued, and the Mediterranean, MIND, and AHEI diets similarly affect metabolomic biomarkers (Tanaka et al., 2022), which other researchers have also observed. Different dietary patterns have different effects on many metabolites, and he stated that dietary intervention to target any single metabolite is misguided.

Ferrucci shared evidence to demonstrate that for the MIND and AHEI dietary patterns, metabolomic signature strongly mediated the association between dietary pattern and frailty index—60–80 percent of the outcome was driven by metabolomic signatures produced by the intervention diet (Tanaka et al., 2022). These findings are important because they indicate that metabolite presence and levels can be an objective measure of dietary quality.

NATIONAL HEALTH AND NUTRITION
EXAMINATION SURVEY

Shinyoung Jun, National Cancer Center in Korea, shared findings from the NHANES, a nationally representative survey operated by the National Center for Health Statistics (NCHS) at the Centers for Disease Control and Prevention. NHANES has been a continuous program since 1999 and collects cross-sectional data from approximately 5,000 people annually, with a target population of noninstitutionalized, civilian residents in the 50 states and the District of Columbia. Jun explained that the sampling method is a multistage, stratified, clustered design with sampling domains that aim to reliably represent age, sex, income, and race and Hispanic origin subgroups.

Jun described NHANES' extensive data collection methods. Participants first complete an in-home interview during which they provide sociodemographic information, disclose any medical conditions, and answer questions about diet behaviors and food security and food assistance program participation. They also provide containers and labels for any dietary supplements used during the past 30 days, along with the frequency, dose, and amount of each. During a second phase of data collection, participants complete a physical examination at the NHANES mobile examination center that includes body measurements, a blood draw, clinical examinations, and a 24-hour dietary recall. A second 24-hour dietary recall is collected by telephone 3–10 days later. Both recalls query participants about intake of foods, beverages, and dietary supplements. Jun explained that dietary data processing begins when NHANES interviewers type responses into computers for direct transmission to NCHS databases, where coders process the data into information about dietary supplement use and food and beverage consumption. Dietary supplement use is converted to nutrient intake from supplements using the NHANES dietary supplement database, and food and beverage consumption is converted to nutrient intakes using the U.S. Department of Agriculture (USDA) Food and Nutrition Database for Dietary Studies.

Dietary supplement use is high among older adults (60+ years old), with the majority using at least one (Figure 2-4). Most supplement users reported multiple products, with the most common being multivitamin and minerals, vitamin D, omega-3, B-complexes, calcium and vitamin D, and vitamin C (Gahche et al., 2017).

Jun stated that when only foods and beverages (and not dietary supplements) are considered, dietary quality (as measured by adherence to the Healthy Eating Index [HEI]) is generally low. Her team's assessment of nutrition status by body weight status among older adults (≥60 years of age) who completed both 24-hour dietary recalls for NHANES found that the mean HEI scores were lower among those with obesity (body mass

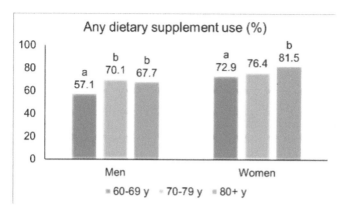

FIGURE 2-4 Any dietary supplement use among older adults (≥60 years of age) in NHANES 2011–2014.
NOTE: Letters (a) and (b) at the top of the columns indicate significant differences from each other.
SOURCE: Presented by Shinyoung Jun on April 8, 2022 (Gahche et al., 2017).

index [BMI] ≥30 kg/m²) than those at a healthy weight (BMI 18.5–24.9 kg/m²) (Figure 2-5).

Jun pointed out that a strength of NHANES is that total usual nutrient intake estimation (from both dietary supplements and foods and beverages) is possible: "usual nutrient intake" is a long-term, average intake that can be compared to recommended levels, such as the dietary reference intakes, and "total usual nutrient intake" is the usual intakes from both diet (foods and beverages) and supplements. Long-term intake is difficult to measure, but can be estimated from short-term measures by applying statistical techniques. At least one 24-hour recall from all participants and a second 24-hour recall from a subsample is needed to derive usual nutrient intake from diet, and a combination of a 30-day dietary supplement frequency questionnaire plus the two 24-hour recalls may be the ideal way to capture usual nutrient intake from dietary supplements (Bailey et al., 2019; Cowan et al., 2020).

Jun shared her research estimating total usual intake for several nutrients designated as underconsumed by the Dietary Guidelines for Americans. Many older adults were found to be at risk of inadequate intake for several of those (which include calcium, magnesium, zinc, folate, vitamin B6, vitamin B12, vitamin C, and vitamin D), but including dietary supplements considerably reduced the proportion of those at risk (Jun et al., 2020). Jun noted that women who had obesity had a higher risk of inadequacy for calcium, magnesium, vitamin B6, and vitamin D (as did men with obesity,

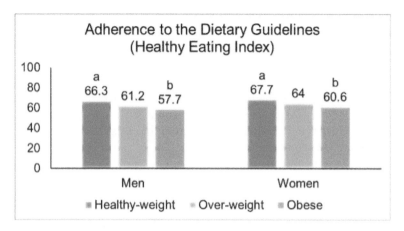

FIGURE 2-5 Adherence to the Dietary Guidelines for Americans among male and female older adults (≥60 years of age), National Health and Nutrition Examination Survey 2011–2014.
SOURCE: Presented by Shinyoung Jun on April 8, 2022 (Jun et al., 2020).

for magnesium) compared with women who had a healthy weight. This finding implies that obesity may coexist with micronutrient inadequacy, despite a common assumption that people with obesity have adequate or excessive food intakes and thus must have adequate micronutrient intake.

Another finding from the same research, Jun continued, was that health risks may cluster in certain population subgroups. About 40 percent of U.S. older adults have obesity, and in addition to the coexistence of obesity with lower dietary quality and micronutrient inadequacy, other risks included self-reported fair or poor overall health, five or more prescription medications used, limitations in activities of daily living, metabolic risk factors, osteoporosis, and participation in the Supplemental Nutrition Assistance Program (SNAP).

Jun listed challenges of using NHANES dietary data, which are cross-sectional and thus lacking temporality. In her view, the biggest challenge is that the data are self-reported and therefore subject to recall bias, which might become magnified among older adults who are experiencing cognitive decline. Proxy reporters may supplement a respondent's reporting, but that has its own limitations. Jun highlighted that data from participants older than 80 are top-coded for privacy, which makes characterizing the "oldest old" challenging. In addition, NHANES targets noninstitutionalized older adults and requires participants to come to the mobile examination center, which may attract a relatively healthy older adult population. Another challenge is the need to regularly update the dietary supplement database to keep pace with the dynamic market for these products.

Jun ended by listing strengths of the NHANES dietary data collection methods. Its ability to produce nationally representative estimates makes it suitable for informing health policy and programs, and the wealth of sociodemographic and health information collected can enable identification of vulnerable subgroups. In-home interview in tandem with a product inventory for dietary supplement intake is a useful method to reduce recall bias, because interviewers check the labels and bottles. Recall bias can also be addressed by use of biomarkers, whereby blood and urine samples are used to produce biomarker information that may calibrate self-reported dietary intake if the nutrient of interest has a potential or known biomarker.

NATIONAL HEALTH AND AGING TRENDS STUDY

Rose Ann DiMaria-Ghalili, Drexel University, explained how her research team used data from the NHATS to produce robust estimates of malnutrition in community-dwelling older adults at a national level. She began by stating that older adults are at risk for malnutrition due to contributors such as physiological changes associated with aging, medications, dietary changes, social conditions, economic factors, and chronic health conditions. In hospitals, malnutrition or nutrition risk affects 12–72 percent of older adults depending on diagnostic criteria used, and some larger datasets of U.S. inpatient samples indicate that patients coded for malnutrition in this setting tend to be 65 and older and have greater infection rates, lengths of stay, costs, and morbidity and mortality rates. Older adults with a malnutrition diagnosis are more likely to be admitted to the hospital from and to be discharged to a skilled nursing facility (Corkins et al., 2014; DiMaria-Ghalili and Nicolo, 2014, p. 3; Heersink et al., 2010).

Turning to the prevalence of malnutrition among U.S. community-dwelling older adults, DiMaria-Ghalili said that gaps remained because a nationally representative sample with this information is not known. About a decade ago, data were collected using an adapted Mini Nutritional Assessment (MNA) as part of the Southeast Pennsylvania Household Health Survey, and 6 percent of such adults were malnourished and 54 percent were at risk (DiMaria-Ghalili et al., 2013). An opportunity to obtain such information on a national level became available in the years following, she said, by conducting a secondary analysis of the NHATS longitudinal cohort.

DiMaria-Ghalili provided a brief overview of the NHATS study, funded by the National Institute on Aging, which is a nationally representative sample of Medicare beneficiaries 65+ that began in 2011 to study late-life disability trends and trajectories. Participants complete in-person assessments and answer questions about medical, social, functional, and technology domains. NHATS collected dried blood samples containing inflammatory biomarkers during its seventh round of data collection in 2017, which her group obtained special permission to use.

To explain how her team assessed malnutrition among NHATS participants, DiMaria-Ghalili recapped the six topics assessed in the MNA:[2] food intake, weight loss, mobility, psychological stress or acute disease, neuropsychological problems (dementia or depression), and BMI. She explained that her group identified items in the NHATS survey that aligned with the MNA, which allowed them to construct a derived MNA from the survey data. The resulting MNA screening score could calculate derived nutrition status score: 12–14 points is normal, 8–11 points is at risk for malnutrition, and 0–7 points is malnourished (Guigoz, 2006; Kaiser et al., 2009; Rubenstein et al., 2001; Vellas et al., 2006). The research team also examined other variables, such as sociodemographic factors (gender, age, living arrangement), health status (self-rated health, chronic conditions, falls, hospitalization), food security, and inflammation.

DiMaria-Ghalili discussed the research sample size and findings: 4,472 participants were included, after exclusion based on factors such as living in a nursing home. After applying weights to the sample, it represents 31 million U.S. older adults in 2017. Based on the MNA-derived screening score, 68 percent were normal, 26 percent were at risk for malnutrition, and about 6 percent were malnourished. DiMaria-Ghalili elaborated on characteristics of participants who were more likely to have malnutrition, which she said included older age (relative to the sample), female gender, living alone in the community, and living in (non-nursing-home) residential care, such as assisted living. No difference was observed by race or ethnicity.

Findings were also stratified by self-reported health-related variables, which indicated that individuals with malnutrition were more likely to self-report their health as fair or poor, have more chronic conditions, and report both falls and hospitalizations in the past year. These results are consistent with findings about malnutrition risk factors among older adults. When nutritional status was examined by food security, individuals with malnutrition were more likely to use Meals on Wheels but no differences in nutrition status were observed based on other food security questions, such as skipping meals due to lack of money or participating in federal food assistance programs.

DiMaria-Ghalili highlighted her study's assessment of inflammatory markers and malnutrition, noting that a reason for heightened interest in diagnosing malnutrition is based on the inflammatory aspects of the condition. NHATS collected two biomarkers of inflammation, C-reactive protein (hsCRP) and interleukin-6 (IL-6), via dried blood samples. These specimens made it possible for the research team to calculate that compared

---

[2] www.mna-elderly.com (accessed September 14, 2022).

with individuals with normal nutrition status, individuals with malnutrition were more likely to have hsCRP levels above the median, and those at nutritional risk were more likely to have IL-6 levels above the median. In other words, older adults who have or are at risk for malnutrition also have inflammation.

DiMaria-Ghalili shared a few conclusions. Despite the limitation of deriving nutrition status based on NHATS items mapped to the MNA, the study's results indicate that malnutrition is not limited to the hospital setting and that an interrelationship exists between malnutrition and inflammation in older adults. She espoused interdisciplinary approaches to address malnutrition in community-dwelling older adults to promote healthy aging and suggested that future work examine the impact of malnutrition on health outcomes and relationship to physical performance.

THE LONGITUDINAL AGING STUDY AMSTERDAM

Marjolein Visser, Vrije Universiteit Amsterdam, discussed assessment of dietary intake in older adults participating in the LASA. This nationally representative sample from the Netherlands includes more than 5,000 participants and uses a multidisciplinary approach that focuses on physical, cognitive, psychological, and social aging over time. The first cohort of approximately 3,100 people was recruited in 1992, and a new cohort of approximately 1,000 people has been added to enrich the sample every 10 years (in 2002 and 2012) as well as a migrant cohort (in 2013) of the first generation of Turkish and Moroccan people in the Netherlands (Hoogendijk et al., 2016, 2020; Huisman et al., 2011). Visser recounted that nutritional status was an area of focus from the beginning, but dietary assessment was not performed until 2014–2015. The resulting data have been used to examine a number of relationships, such as dietary patterns and depression, protein intake and functional outcomes and sarcopenia, and dietary protein intake and overall diet sustainability.

Visser explained that individuals in the study were invited to participate in ancillary studies—more than 1,400 out of approximately 2,000 eligible individuals completed an FFQ. This response rate of 68.9 percent was higher than the response rate in the national dietary survey, and she attributed nonresponses to people who are either very frail or relatively young, active, and short on time. The FFQ was offered on paper or digitally, she said, and about half of the sample completed it online. The online questionnaires had fewer missing data than the paper questionnaires, Visser added, because respondents skipped pages on the latter.

She described the FFQ, which queried respondents on frequencies and portion sizes of nearly 240 food items during the prior 4 weeks. Participants could indicate consumption amounts using standard units (e.g., slices of bread) and household units (e.g., tablespoons) and by selecting pictures that represented their typical consumption. She explained that question-naires were excluded if they had missing items or reported implausibly high energy intakes. However, those with implausibly low energy intakes were not excluded, as is often done with FFQs. This decision was made because the 24-hour recall data for a subset of participants indicated that many older people have habitually low energy intakes. The 24-hour recall data were available because some participants who completed the FFQ were selected for three 24-hour recalls as part of a validation study. The FFQ was developed for a wide age range, so the researchers wanted to assess whether it would also be valid in a sample comprised exclusively of older people.

Visser shared the methodology for the three 24-hour recalls; two were performed on weekdays and the third on a weekend. Prior to the first recall, participants received information about best practices for measuring food quantities using frequently used kitchenware and a picture book with por-tion sizes. During the interviews—which were unscheduled so as not to influence intake on the interview day—interviewers asked participants to reference the picture book. Eighty-eight individuals with an average age of 71.9 were included in the sample, which was deemed sufficiently representa-tive of the total FFQ sample (Visser et al., 2020).

Visser discussed the validation results for macronutrients, a selection of micronutrients, and a selection of food groups. For energy and mac-ronutrients, the group-level bias was small, and the quintile agreement was moderate to high (i.e., most individuals were ranked in the same or adjacent quintiles of intake on both the FFQ and the 24-hour recall). For most micronutrients and food groups, the Pearson's correlation coefficients were moderate, and for all the micronutrients and most food groups, quin-tile agreement was moderate to high. An exception was legumes and fish because the FFQ overestimated intake of those food groups and they are not well captured in 24-hour dietary recalls due to infrequent consumption and low daily intake.

Relative to other Dutch FFQ validation studies conducted in younger adults, Visser indicated similar or only slightly lower Pearson's correlations. This suggests that FFQs are as valid in older adults, and the validity of the FFQ is similar to that of FFQs in older adults from other countries. She also noted that conducting 24-hour recalls by phone is less affected by the participant's visual or physical limitations as compared with an FFQ.

Visser shared the study's methods for assessing dietary supplement intake. In several survey waves, specific supplement use was queried via interviewer-administered questions at home. This led to suboptimal record-ing of information, such as failure to report specific vitamins, such as vitamin D, that were part of multivitamin supplements. In more recent waves of the survey, all dietary supplements were recorded in the same way as medication use (participants provided all bottles and containers of prescribed and nonprescribed supplements used during the past 2 weeks, and interviewers recorded label information [brand name, dose, concentration, etc.]). It would seem that this method easily lends itself to calculating intake of nutrients through supplements, but it is more challenging than it may seem. Despite an annual updating of the Dutch Supplement Database with new brands, labels, and concentrations, it is still a challenge to obtain their true intake. As true dietary supplements are often not included in the database, people may face difficulty or make errors when inputting them. This challenge led Visser's team to develop an algorithm to ensure the best estimate of nutrient intake from dietary supplements among older adults (Figure 2-6).

PANEL DISCUSSION WITH SPEAKERS

Following the six presentations, speakers answered questions from the workshop planning committee and attendees about a variety of topics related to dietary assessment of older adults: using biological specimens to assess dietary intake, assessing and addressing inflammation, assessing supplement use, stratifying cohorts by age beyond 80 years, using technology, issues associated with clinical populations, priority metrics to collect in clinical settings, and vision for future dietary assessment practices.

Using Biological Specimens to Assess Dietary Intake

In response to a question about the utility of biological specimens for enhancing dietary assessment methods, Ferrucci stated that the science of evaluating dietary intake through biomarkers is advancing. He encouraged routine use of biomarker data, such as metabolomic assessment reports, in clinical settings to evaluate dietary quality of older adults. The costs could be reasonable if done at a large scale, and collecting objective markers of intake would be less burdensome on providers and patients than asking them to complete traditional dietary assessment instruments. DiMaria-Ghalili urged consideration of how to bridge the gap of what is feasible in research settings versus clinical practice, noting that advances in knowledge and tools are gradually broadening the scope of what is possible in health care settings. Visser added that different assessment methods and biomarkers are needed to produce estimates of how well an individual's diet aligns with recommended dietary patterns versus intake of single nutrients, to which Regan Bailey, session moderator, commented that triangulating

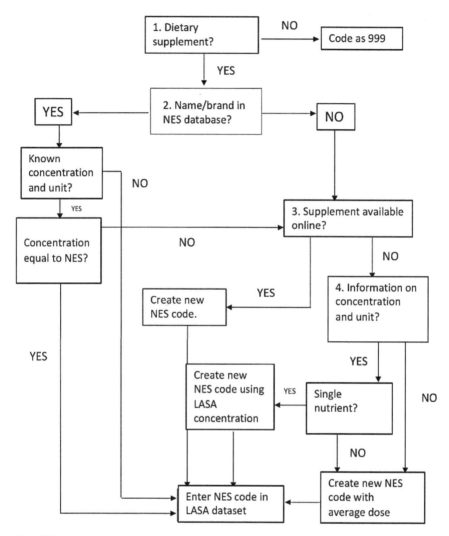

FIGURE 2-6 Algorithm to optimize estimating nutrient intake from dietary supplements among older adults.
NOTE: NES = Dutch supplement database; LASA = Longitudinal Aging Study Amsterdam.
SOURCE: Presented by Marjolein Visser on April 8, 2022.

exposure from several complementary methods of assessment is a viable approach.

Assessing and Addressing Inflammation

Another question related to biomarkers was how to consider inflammation when assessing dietary intakes of older adults, given its effect on nutrient digestion and absorption. Ferrucci emphasized that inflammatory status is affected by diet and physical activity, stress, and other factors, and despite accumulation of high-quality evidence about inflammatory biomarkers and their relationship to health outcomes, they are rarely measured in practice. He urged researchers to consider how inflammation—chronic or acute—might affect older adults' nutritional requirements, referencing the increased protein requirement in the context of high inflammation due to its effects on muscle protein synthesis. Jun agreed, suggesting that because dietary reference intakes are designed for healthy people, they may need to be revised (evidence permitting) for the many individuals with multiple chronic conditions that promote an inflammatory state. Volkert added that because inflammation impairs appetite, it is important to identify strategies to improve food intake. Ferrucci raised the possibility of dietary strategies to block inflammation and ensuing disease, urging research to identify nutrition interventions.

Assessing Supplement Use

Visser replied to a question about strategies to assess supplement use in older adults; open-ended recall via questionnaire is much less effective than asking participants to provide the actual bottles. Researchers can then query participants about dose and copy information from the label about brand, nutrient content, and ingredients (this information may also be contained in databases used for dietary assessment studies), although she cautioned that label (or database) information may not always match the actual contents due to factors such as deterioration over time or changes in formulation without updates to the label (or database).

Stratifying Cohorts by Age Beyond 80 Years

A workshop participant asked about the value of separating study cohorts into further age-defined subgroups after 80 to observe differences in health outcomes DiMaria-Ghalili confirmed that NHATS data are available for individuals over 80 and could be stratified beyond that point, but for NHATS and other studies, some of these data may be restricted and less accessible for analysis. Keller shared that examining cohorts by 5-year age subgroups (e.g., 80–85, 86–90) could help focus analysis and might be considered moving forward.

Using Technology

Keller recalled Visser's comment about the positive uptake of a digitally based FFQ in one of her studies and asked what advice she would give to others interested in using technology for dietary assessment of older adults. Visser elaborated that half of participants voluntarily opted to complete the FFQ digitally, which she attributed to a high prevalence of Internet use in the Netherlands across socioeconomic groups. She urged others to consider rates of Internet use by demographic groups in a study's geographic area, lest results be biased by different rates in certain age or income groups, for example.

Issues Associated with Clinical Populations

Keller asked the speakers to consider approaches to improve dietary assessment in clinical populations, which are vulnerable to malnutrition and frailty. Ferrucci raised the issue of anorexia among aging clinical populations, stating that low food intake and appetite, along with declining weight, is often associated with depression. He suggested that assessment tools consider anorexia and its risk factors, including those that might seem trivial, such as the ability to chew and swallow easily. Visser called attention to the seemingly opposite issue of obesity in older adults, which she said is often overlooked and also often associated with low protein intake. Volkert added that the ability to self-report food intake depends on cognitive ability, physical status, and frailty status, and she wondered if research had examined the validity of dietary assessment in the oldest old (>80) in residential settings. Bailey and Jun pointed out that NHANES has a subset of participants 80 and older, which they thought could be compared to older adults in the 60- and 70-year ranges. DiMaria-Ghalili suggested that waves of data collection with U.S. longitudinal cohorts incorporate nutrition measures to generate standardized measures across study populations.

Priority Metrics to Collect in Clinical Settings

Ferrucci responded to a related question about which metrics should be prioritized for collection in clinical settings, remarking that this question is "enormously complex." He observed that free-living older adult populations have been more well studied than those in nursing homes or residential assisted-living facilities, which vary widely in how they are operated. Researchers and clinicians could contact the people who care directly for residents in those facilities to understand how things work there and what questions should be part of a dietary assessment. He urged a continued focus on disease prevention through good nutrition and attention to existing problems, such as anorexia. Volkert provided a list of measures to assess, including appetite (i.e., desire to eat), weight, and recent weight history. DiMaria-Ghalili suggested that because of the overlap among common conditions in older adults (e.g., malnutrition, sarcopenia, frailty, cachexia), it may be helpful to use an appropriate metric to help differentiate conditions so that intervention and treatment can be provided accordingly (noting that some treatments may be suitable to address more than one condition). Visser mentioned that body weight is often monitored at nursing homes in the Netherlands to watch for malnutrition, but measures of diet quality, such as fruit and vegetable intake, are important but rarely collected. Keller shared that in her experience assessing food intake in long-term care populations, more than half of participants did not meet dietary intake recommendations for one-third of vitamins assessed (Keller et al., 2018). Lack of knowledge may be part of the problem, Visser suggested, referencing her research that indicated unawareness among older adults of protein sources (e.g., one-third of the sample thought that tomato contained more protein than an equivalent weight of beef) and recommended intake amounts (e.g., many people in the sample thought that one meal per day with a good protein source was adequate) (Visser et al., 2021).

Opportunities for Future Dietary Assessment Practices

The final question asked speakers to describe one change they would like to see in nutrition assessment for older adults. DiMaria-Ghalili said she would like nutrition screening or assessment to be added to the Medicare annual wellness exam. In Ferrucci's dream world, people would think about and recognize how their current dietary choices shape their future health and experiences; young people tend to think that their food choices do not matter, but evidence indicates that early life choices accumulate to have an impact on health and disease as one ages. Visser agreed and added that she would want people to realize that it is never too late to adopt healthier eating habits and that doing so has immediate benefits. Jun imagined that technological advances in assessment methods, such as image-based approaches, could greatly reduce the burden of current methods. A newer approach that Visser said she would like to see expanded is a version of ecological momentary assessment, whereby participants receive messages in an app at random times of the day for weeks and are prompted to enter what they consumed in the past hour. This is a relatively low-burden approach, with satisfactory validity data.

REFERENCES

Bailey, R. L., K. W. Dodd, J. J. Gahche, J. T. Dwyer, A. E. Cowan, S. Jun, H. A. Eicher-Miller, P. M. Guenther, A. Bhadra, P. R. Thomas, N. Potischman, R. J. Carroll, and J. A. Tooze. 2019. Best practices for dietary supplement assessment and estimation of total usual nutrient intakes in population-level research and monitoring. *Journal of Nutrition* 149(2):181–197.

Bohne, S. E. J., M. Hiesmayr, I. Sulz, S. Tarantino, R. Wirth, and D. Volkert. 2022. Recent and current low food intake—prevalence and associated factors in hospital patients from different medical specialities. *European Journal of Clinical Nutrition* 76(10):1440–1448.

Buettner, D., and S. Skemp. 2016. Blue zones: Lessons from the world's longest lived. *American Journal of Lifestyle Medicine* 10(5):318–321.

Corkins, M. R., P. Guenter, R. A. DiMaria-Ghalili, G. L. Jensen, A. Malone, S. Miller, V. Patel, S. Plogsted, H. E. Resnick, and American Society for Parenteral and Enteral Nutrition. 2014. Malnutrition diagnoses in hospitalized patients: United States, 2010. *Journal of Parenteral and Enteral Nutrition* 38(2):186–195.

Cowan, A. E., S. Jun, J. A. Tooze, K. W. Dodd, J. J. Gahche, H. A. Eicher-Miller, P. M. Guenther, J. T. Dwyer, A. J. Moshfegh, D. G. Rhodes, A. Bhadra, and R. L. Bailey. 2020. Comparison of 4 methods to assess the prevalence of use and estimates of nutrient intakes from dietary supplements among U.S. adults. *Journal of Nutrition* 150(4):884–893.

DiMaria-Ghalili, R. A., Y. L. Michael, and A. L. Rosso. 2013. Malnutrition in a sample of community-dwelling older Pennsylvanians. *Journal of Aging Research & Clinical Practice* 2(1):39–45.

DiMaria-Ghalili, R. A., and M. Nicolo. 2014. Nutrition and hydration in older adults in critical care. *Critical Care Nursing Clinics of North America* 26(1):31–45.

Gahche, J. J., R. L. Bailey, N. Potischman, and J. T. Dwyer. 2017. Dietary supplement use was very high among older adults in the United States in 2011–2014. *Journal of Nutrition* 147(10):1968–1976.

Guigoz, Y. 2006. The Mini Nutritional Assessment (MNA) review of the literature—what does it tell us? *Journal of Nutrition, Health & Aging* 10(6):466–485; discussion 485–487.

Heersink, J. T., C. J. Brown, R. A. DiMaria-Ghalili, and J. L. Locher. 2010. Undernutrition in hospitalized older adults: Patterns and correlates, outcomes, and opportunities for intervention with a focus on processes of care. *Journal of Nutrition for the Elderly* 29(1):4–41.

Hoogendijk, E. O., D. J. Deeg, J. Poppelaars, M. van der Horst, M. I. Broese van Groenou, H. C. Comijs, H. R. Pasman, N. M. van Schoor, B. Suanet, F. Thomese, T. G. van Tilburg, M. Visser, and M. Huisman. 2016. The Longitudinal Aging Study Amsterdam: Cohort update 2016 and major findings. *European Journal of Epidemiology* 31(9):927–945.

Hoogendijk, E. O., D. J. H. Deeg, S. de Breij, S. S. Klokgieters, A. A. L. Kok, N. Stringa, E. J. Timmermans, N. M. van Schoor, E. M. van Zutphen, M. van der Horst, J. Poppelaars, P. Malhoe, and M. Huisman. 2020. The Longitudinal Aging Study Amsterdam: Cohort update 2019 and additional data collections. *European Journal of Epidemiology* 35(1):61–74.

Huisman, M., J. Poppelaars, M. van der Horst, A. T. Beekman, J. Brug, T. G. van Tilburg, and D. J. Deeg. 2011. Cohort profile: The Longitudinal Aging Study Amsterdam. *International Journal of Epidemiology* 40(4):868–876.

Jun, S., A. E. Cowan, A. Bhadra, K. W. Dodd, J. T. Dwyer, H. A. Eicher-Miller, J. J. Gahche, P. M. Guenther, N. Potischman, J. A. Tooze, and R. L. Bailey. 2020. Older adults with obesity have higher risks of some micronutrient inadequacies and lower overall dietary quality compared to peers with a healthy weight, National Health and Nutrition Examination Surveys (NHANES), 2011–2014. *Public Health Nutrition* 23(13):2268–2279.

Kaiser, M. J., J. M. Bauer, C. Ramsch, W. Uter, Y. Guigoz, T. Cederholm, D. R. Thomas, P. Anthony, K. E. Charlton, M. Maggio, A. C. Tsai, D. Grathwohl, B. Vellas, C. C. Sieber, and M. N. A.-International Group. 2009. Validation of the Mini Nutritional Assessment Short-Form (MNA-SF): A practical tool for identification of nutritional status. *Journal of Nutrition, Health & Aging* 13(9):782–788.

Keller, H. H., C. Lengyel, N. Carrier, S. E. Slaughter, J. Morrison, A. M. Duncan, C. M. Steele, L. Duizer, K. S. Brown, H. Chaudhury, M. N. Yoon, V. Boscart, G. Heckman, and L. Villalon. 2018. Prevalence of inadequate micronutrient intakes of Canadian long-term care residents. *British Journal of Nutrition* 119(9):1047–1056.

Milaneschi, Y., S. Bandinelli, A. M. Corsi, F. Lauretani, G. Paolisso, L. J. Dominguez, R. D. Semba, T. Tanaka, A. M. Abbatecola, S. A. Talegawkar, J. M. Guralnik, and L. Ferrucci. 2011. Mediterranean diet and mobility decline in older persons. *Experimental Gerontology* 46(4):303–308.

Quach, A., M. E. Levine, T. Tanaka, A. T. Lu, B. H. Chen, L. Ferrucci, B. Ritz, S. Bandinelli, M. L. Neuhouser, J. M. Beasley, L. Snetselaar, R. B. Wallace, P. S. Tsao, D. Absher, T. L. Assimes, J. D. Stewart, Y. Li, L. Hou, A. A. Baccarelli, E. A. Whitsel, and S. Horvath. 2017. Epigenetic clock analysis of diet, exercise, education, and lifestyle factors. *Aging* 9(2):419–446.

Rubenstein, L. Z., J. O. Harker, A. Salva, Y. Guigoz, and B. Vellas. 2001. Screening for undernutrition in geriatric practice: Developing the Short-Form Mini-Nutritional Assessment (MNA-SF). *Journals of Gerontology, Series A, Biological Sciences and Medical Sciences* 56(6):M366–372.

Schindler, K., M. Themessl-Huber, M. Hiesmayr, S. Kosak, M. Lainscak, A. Laviano, O. Ljungqvist, M. Mouhieddine, S. Schneider, M. de van der Schueren, T. Schutz, C. Schuh, P. Singer, P. Bauer, and C. Pichard. 2016. To eat or not to eat? Indicators for reduced food intake in 91,245 patients hospitalized on nutritionDays 2006–2014 in 56 countries worldwide: A descriptive analysis. *American Journal of Clinical Nutrition* 104(5):1393–1402.

Talegawkar, S. A., S. Bandinelli, K. Bandeen-Roche, P. Chen, Y. Milaneschi, T. Tanaka, R. D. Semba, J. M. Guralnik, and L. Ferrucci. 2012. A higher adherence to a Mediterranean-style diet is inversely associated with the development of frailty in community-dwelling elderly men and women. *Journal of Nutrition* 142(12):2161–2166.

Talegawkar, S. A., Y. Jin, E. M. Simonsick, K. L. Tucker, L. Ferrucci, and T. Tanaka. 2022. The Mediterranean-DASH Intervention for Neurodegenerative Delay (MIND) diet is associated with physical function and grip strength in older men and women. *American Journal of Clinical Nutrition* 115(3):625–632.

Tanaka, T., S. A. Talegawkar, Y. Jin, M. Colpo, L. Ferrucci, and S. Bandinelli. 2018. Adherence to a Mediterranean diet protects from cognitive decline in the Invecchiare in Chianti study of aging. *Nutrients* 10(12).

Tanaka, T., S. A. Talegawkar, Y. Jin, S. Bandinelli, and L. Ferrucci. 2021. Association of adherence to the Mediterranean-style diet with lower frailty index in older adults. *Nutrients* 13(4).

Tanaka, T., S. A. Talegawkar, Y. Jin, J. Candia, Q. Tian, R. Moaddel, E. M. Simonsick, and L. Ferrucci. 2022. Metabolomic profile of different dietary patterns and their association with frailty index in community-dwelling older men and women. *Nutrients* 14(11).

Tarantino, S., M. Hiesmayr, I. Sulz, and nDay Working Group. 2022. NutritionDay worldwide annual report 2019. *Clinical Nutrition ESPEN* 49:560–667.

UN (United Nations) DESA Population Division. 2019. *World population prospects 2019*. https://population.un.org/wpp/publications/files/wpp2019_highlights.pdf (accessed September 14, 2022).

Vellas, B., H. Villars, G. Abellan, M. E. Soto, Y. Rolland, Y. Guigoz, J. E. Morley, W. Chumlea, A. Salva, L. Z. Rubenstein, and P. Garry. 2006. Overview of the MNA—its history and challenges. *Journal of Nutrition, Health & Aging* 10(6):456–463; discussion 463–465.

Visser, M., L. E. M. Elstgeest, L. H. H. Winkens, I. A. Brouwer, and M. Nicolaou. 2020. Relative validity of the Helius Food Frequency Questionnaire for measuring dietary intake in older adult participants of the Longitudinal Aging Study Amsterdam. *Nutrients* 12(7).

Visser, M., Y. Hung, and W. Verbeke. 2021. Protein knowledge of older adults and identification of subgroups with poor knowledge. *Nutrients* 13(3).

WHO (World Health Organization). 2021. *Decade of healthy ageing: Baseline report.*

Zamora-Ros, R., M. Rabassa, A. Cherubini, M. Urpi-Sarda, S. Bandinelli, L. Ferrucci, and C. Andres-Lacueva. 2013. High concentrations of a urinary biomarker of polyphenol intake are associated with decreased mortality in older adults. *Journal of Nutrition* 143(9):1445–1450.

3

Advances and Key Issues in Dietary Assessment of Older Adults

BOX 3-1
Highlights[a]

- The Geisinger Rural Aging Study (GRAS) cohort has a high prevalence of poor-quality diets, obesity, and poor health. Now in its third decade of data collection, the study has concluded that telephone dietary recalls remain a gold standard for quantifying nutrient and food intake in older adults. Throughout GRAS, a brief dietary screening tool was developed and validated as an effective measure of risk for inadequate dietary intake and poor diet quality in older adults; validation in more diverse populations would broaden its reach. (Mitchell)
- According to the Georgia Centenarian Study, this population has a high prevalence of poor vitamin D and vitamin B12 status, but that can be improved with supplement use. Docosahexaenoic acid (DHA), lutein, and zeaxanthin appear to be positively correlated with cognition and brain health, and large ranges in concentrations of these biomarkers in blood and brain tissue suggest persistent responsiveness to nutrition late in life. (Johnson)
- Dutch experiences with dietary assessment of older adults suggest that 24-hour recalls and food frequency questionnaires (FFQs) are as effective for older people as they are for younger people. Assessment tools would benefit from further validation, particularly in lower socioeconomic populations; methods and tools could be refined by investigating the relationship between cognitive capabilities (cognition, vision, hearing, writing ability) and/or overall physical functionality and accurate reporting in diverse older adult populations. (Jeanne de Vries)

- Dietary recall methods allow open-ended capture of diverse diets and are useful for describing distributions of populations but not usual intake. FFQs are useful for ranking groups and predicting health outcomes but can produce substantial bias in multicultural studies due to their inability to equally represent diets of different groups. Strategies exist for adapting existing FFQs for different ethnic/cultural or regional populations; these methods are neither simple nor inexpensive but are critical for improving the validity of intake data for diverse populations. (Tucker)
- Smartphone ownership and Internet usage is on the rise among older adults, many of whom have compatible devices for downloading health-related apps and appear to be willing to do so. Evidence suggests that older adults are compliant with either self- or interview-administered automated 24-hour recall tools; such methods and other technology-assisted approaches to measure dietary intake must be informed by research to assess how they can advance dietary assessment of older adults. (Fialkowski Revilla)

---

*a*This list is the rapporteurs' summary of points made by the individual speakers identified, and the statements have not been endorsed or verified by the National Academies of Sciences, Engineering, and Medicine. They are not intended to reflect a consensus among workshop participants.

The second workshop, held April 22, 2022, featured five presentations about advances and key issues in dietary assessment of older adults, followed by a panel discussion with the speakers. These topics were explored through case studies and examples from a variety of longitudinal cohorts that have assessed dietary intakes among older adults. Diane C. Mitchell, Penn State University, and Carol Boushey, University of Hawai'i Cancer Center and chair of the workshop planning committee, moderated the second workshop.

ASSESSING NUTRITION RISK AMONG COMMUNITY-DWELLING RURAL OLDER ADULTS: THE GEISINGER RURAL AGING STUDY

Mitchell introduced the second workshop's topic and discussed the application and development of methods used in the Geisinger Rural Aging Study (GRAS)[1] and the effectiveness of a brief assessment tool for use in this cohort. She reiterated the importance of developing more feasible, valid, and reliable dietary assessment methods for older adults given the rapidly

---

[1] https://portal.nifa.usda.gov/web/crisprojectpages/0427231-rural-aging-study-geisinger.html (accessed September 14, 2022).

aging global population with a high prevalence of obesity, malnutrition, and poor eating habits.

Mitchell began with a description of the GRAS cohort, which was recruited from a pool of more than two million people in central Pennsylvania, a mostly rural area where the leading industry is agriculture. This population is largely White, native to Pennsylvania, and sparse (population density of 14–475 people per square mile), with greater than 20 percent of residents in many counties aged 60 years and older. The Geisinger Healthcare System service area has one of the largest U.S. concentrations of rural older persons, and it implemented a regional nutrition screening program in 1994 that targeted all members in a Medicare risk contract. It enrolled participants through 1999, which established the GRAS cohort.

Mitchell elaborated on the screening process, which occurred in baseline clinic visits. After enrollment, participants were screened using a one-page questionnaire that was slightly modified from the original Level I and II nutrition screening questionnaires developed in the early 1990s. The screening initiative resulted in a GRAS cohort of 21,645 older adults outside of assisted living (community-dwelling adults) (Bailey et al., 2007, p. 12).

Mitchell explained that the GRAS objectives—to characterize dietary patterns and examine relationships between nutrition risk and health outcomes, including BMI, quality of life, diet quality, various comorbidities (cardiovascular disease, diabetes, hypertension), and mortality—have remained consistent during the study's nearly 25 years. Researchers plan to add variables collected at baseline, to study food insecurity and neurological outcomes. Now in year 3 of the fifth 5-year cycle of data collection, the study has only 15–25 percent of its participants still living, all of whom are 85 or older.

Mitchell provided a high-level overview of the GRAS methodology. Follow-up screening questionnaires were mailed to participants every 3–4 years, and a more specific tool (Dietary Screening Tool [DST]) was added in the 2009 wave of rescreening. Since the early 2000s, researchers have been able to access deidentified electronic health record data for the full cohort, and in three sequential cycles, a series of comprehensive diet assessments were conducted with a representative subset.

The comprehensive diet assessments were part of a broader evaluation conducted with each subset, which included an eligibility criterion of an acceptable score on the Mini-Mental State Exam (MMSE),[2] a test for cognitive ability and geriatric depression using the Geriatric Depression

---

[2] https://www.healthdirect.gov.au/mini-mental-state-examination-mmse#:~:text=about %20the%20MMSE-,What%20is%20a%20Mini%2DMental%20State%20Examination%20 (MMSE)%3F,communication%2C%20understanding%20and%20memory) (accessed September 14, 2022).

32

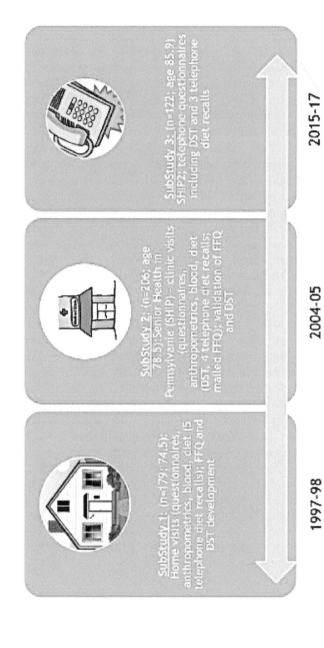

FIGURE 3-1 Comprehensive evaluations in three sequential representative subsets of the GRAS cohort ($n = 21,645$).
SOURCE: Presented by Diane Mitchell on April 22, 2022.

Scale.[3] The first substudy (1997–1998) conducted home visits with 179 participants (average age 74.5) to collect a health questionnaire, anthropometrics, and a blood draw. Next, participants completed five telephone dietary recalls over 1 year (approximately every other month), comprised of unannounced calls on 2 weekend days and 3 weekdays. In addition, an existing food frequency questionnaire (FFQ) was modified and validated for the GRAS population, and a new diet quality questionnaire was developed (the DST). The latter evolved as researchers examined dietary recall data and gradually characterized participants' diets to identify a set of factors and behaviors that could indicate diet quality in the age group represented in GRAS (Bailey et al., 2007). Researchers recognized that the DST would be more feasible, practical, and lower cost for inadequate dietary intake and poor diet quality than traditional methods for assessing diet.

The DST was tested and validated in the second substudy (2004–2005), which included 206 participants (average age 78.5) and was referred to as the "Senior Health in Pennsylvania" study. The DST was administered during clinic visits where research staff also collected height, weight, and other information. A validation process that included comparison with four dietary recalls and nutritional status biomarkers determined that the DST is an effective tool for screening dietary intake; it is the first of its kind to be developed for older adults. Mitchell added that the FFQ was sent and collected via mail—although 75 percent of participants required follow-up telephone calls for incomplete sections—and was validated relative to four unannounced telephone dietary recalls (Mitchell et al., 2012).

The third substudy (2015–2017) included 122 participants (average age 85.9), and all assessments and questionnaires were by telephone. Dietary assessment comprised three dietary recalls and the DST. Mitchell added that the DST has been adapted and used in other populations (Ford et al., 2014; Greene et al., 2018; Jacka et al., 2017; Ventura Marra et al., 2018).

Mitchell presented a comparison of dietary patterns in the first and third substudies, clarifying that each had different participants and slight variation in methods for grouping foods. Cluster analysis was used to generate dietary patterns, which consistently resulted in two distinct patterns (clusters) for both studies: less and more nutrient dense. In both substudies, the less nutrient-dense patterns had higher intakes of desserts and other sweets, for example, and the more nutrient-dense patterns had higher intakes of fruits, vegetables, fish, and eggs.

When nutrient intakes and weight status were examined by dietary pattern in the first substudy, the more nutrient-dense clusters were characterized by higher intakes of protein, fiber, and key vitamins and minerals;

---

[3] https://wwwoundcare.ca/Uploads/ContentDocuments/Geriatric%20Depression%20Scale.pdf (accessed September 14, 2022).

lower intakes of energy and fat; and lower waist circumference (but not body mass index [BMI]). The diets were more homogenous in the third substudy, Mitchell said, but the two patterns were still distinguishable, with the more nutrient-dense cluster characterized by higher intakes of fiber, potassium, and several vitamins, and higher Healthy Eating Index (HEI) and DST scores.

Mitchell summarized key findings from the 23-year duration of research with the GRAS cohort. A high prevalence of poor-quality diets, obesity, and ill health has been observed among the cohort, and GRAS was among the first studies to recognize that obesity in older adults is characterized by poor diet quality, comorbidities, and functional decline. She noted that a poor-quality diet is also associated with low BMI and increased mortality. With respect to the diet assessment methods, telephone dietary recalls remain a gold standard method for quantifying nutrients and foods in older adults despite their limitations (e.g., cost, cognitive issues, and high prevalence of chronic disease that likely influences diet). The GRAS FFQ is a valid assessment of dietary risk as defined by diet quality and poor dietary intake but may not be the best choice for older adults, given the high rate of incomplete assessments returned by participants during the second substudy. Finally, she confirmed that the DST is a valid, brief, and effective screening tool used to measure dietary risk defined by diet quality and nutrient intakes in older adults, but its validity is mostly limited to the GRAS population. Others could follow the GRAS model to develop, test, and validate the DST to create a brief assessment tool for their own populations.

GEORGIA CENTENARIAN STUDY

Mary Ann Johnson, University of Nebraska–Lincoln, shared findings about potentially modifiable risk factors related to nutritional status among participants in the Georgia Centenarian Study. In 2020, it was estimated that 573,000 centenarians live in the world, and the projected figure for 2100 is 19 million (Statista, 2022). Johnson shared her sentiments that it is highly rewarding to study society's oldest individuals, reflecting on an example of a Black centenarian in Atlanta who had been born at a time when women and Black people could not vote and lived to cast her ballot for Barack Obama, the country's first Black president.

The study began in 1988, but the data she presented were collected from 2003 to 2005. The study's objectives are to identify physical, mental, social, nutritional, and genetic factors related to well-being late in life. The cohort is drawn from 44 counties in northeast Georgia: 244 individuals aged 98 and older (the centenarians) and 80 individuals aged 80–89. Participants were identified from skilled nursing facilities, personal care homes, and registered voter lists, and they or their proxies responded to questions and provided informed consent (Poon et al., 2007).

Johnson shared findings on nutrition biomarkers among study participants, beginning with vitamin D. Serum vitamin D was lower in the centenarians than the 80-year-old participants and lower in Black than in White participants, and levels varied by season (highest in fall, lowest in spring) independent of dairy intake and place of residence (facility versus community) (Johnson et al., 2008). Vitamin D insufficiency was 22.5 percent of 80-year-olds and 36.7 percent of the centenarians; 30 percent of White and 61 percent of Black centenarians had insufficiency (Johnson et al., 2008). Prevalence was lower among centenarians who consumed a vitamin-D-containing supplement (20 percent) than those who did not (50 percent) (Johnson et al., 2008). These findings are generally consistent with those of 80+ year-old participants in NHANES III, which was conducted at the same time (Looker et al., 2002). Another study at the time reported undetectable vitamin D levels in 99 of 104 centenarians in northern Italy, but this region is mountainous, cloudy, and rainy, and food fortification and supplement intake were uncommon (Passeri et al., 2003). Johnson summarized that these study results suggest that supplement use is a modifiable risk factor for enhanced vitamin D status among older adults.

Moving on to vitamin B12, Johnson pointed out that the proportion of women, Black or African American individuals, B-vitamin supplement users, and consumers of >2 servings/day of animal foods were similar in both of the study's age groups. Mean serum vitamin B12 was similar in the two age groups (Johnson et al., 2010) and in a Korean cohort where more than 30 percent of vitamin B12 intake was derived from fermented plant foods (Kwak et al., 2010). Vitamin B12 deficiency was significantly higher among the centenarians (35 versus 23 percent) (Johnson et al., 2010), of whom White individuals had a nearly twofold higher B12 deficiency than Black or African American individuals, and supplement use was lower in those who were deficient. Severe atrophic gastritis, which interferes with acid production in the stomach—an intrinsic factor needed for B12 absorption—was significantly more common in the deficient group (Johnson et al., 2010). Johnson reiterated that as with vitamin D, supplement use appears to be a modifiable risk factor for vitamin B12 status, and a culture's dietary patterns also play a role in its aging population's nutrition risk factors.

Johnson described the Georgia Centenarian Study's focus on brain health and the role of nutrients such as docosahexaenoic acid (DHA) and lutein. Thirty-one percent of the centenarian age group agreed to donate their brains to science upon their death (Shaw et al., 2012), and upon examination of the half of the brains without dementia, DHA was the fatty acid category most strongly associated with better scores on 11 of the 14 cognitive tests administered (Mohn et al., 2013). Among centenarians, xanthophylls (i.e., lutein, zeaxanthin, and cryptoxanthin) appear to be preferentially accumulated in the brain compared to the serum (Johnson et al.,

2013), a distribution that may indicate a special function of xanthophylls in the brain. Another study found that lutein and beta-carotene were higher in centenarians with normal cognitive function and lowest in those with mild cognitive impairment (Johnson et al., 2013).

Johnson raised a few limitations of the Georgia Centenarian Study, such as its participant demographic characteristics (e.g., 20 percent Black and 80 percent White), which may limit applicability of the findings to more diverse populations. Supplement intake was also self-reported, often from a proxy reporter.

To summarize key findings, Johnson referenced a high prevalence of poor vitamin D and B12 status, which she called measurable and correctable; a positive association between supplement intake and higher vitamin D and vitamin B12 status; low prevalence of folate deficiency, likely related to U.S. food fortification and relatively widespread supplement use; an apparent positive association of DHA, lutein, and zeaxanthin with cognition and brain health, so the plant sources of these nutrients may be important; and large ranges in the concentrations of these biomarkers in blood and brain tissue, which suggests persistent responsiveness to the nutrition environment even late into life.

IMPLEMENTING DIVERSE DIETARY ASSESSMENT METHODS AMONG COMMUNITY-DWELLING ADULTS OR CLINICAL NURSING HOME RESIDENTS

Jeanne de Vries, Wageningen University, described her experience with applying different dietary assessment tools in the Netherlands' older population. Older adult populations are heterogenous, she began, with a wide age range (60+ to centenarians), physical function (from physically active to fully dependent on care), and degree of mental and physical impairment. She clarified that her studies addressed both healthy and "more fragile" older adults.

With respect to surveillance of dietary intake in older people, de Vries referenced an Efcosum project[4] that raised the need for confirmation of the hypothesis that food intake measurements using retrospective methods would be unsuitable for older people. The project also raised a lack of empirical data indicating that older people face specific problems to completing such dietary assessments. The project added that 24-hour dietary recalls and FFQs may give more accurate information, and accuracy probably depends on the respondent's health status, such that memory deficits

---

[4] https://ec.europa.eu/health/ph_projects/1999/monitoring/fp_monitoring_1999_frep_10_en.pdf (accessed September 14, 2022).

or other physical or cognitive impairments may introduce inaccuracies or challenges completing the assessment.

She summarized highlights from a journal article that recounted experiences from studies to assess dietary intake of older adults in the Netherlands (de Vries et al., 2009), beginning with the Survey in Europe on Nutrition and the Elderly: A Concerted Action longitudinal cohort study. Participants were 75 on average, and researchers were interested in the mean and distribution of usual intake and ranking of intake at the individual level. The method was a modified dietary history (which included a 3-day estimated food record and a dietary history interview) plus a questionnaire that gathered information about food habits and nutrition attitudes. When reported energy and nutrient intakes from the interview were compared with those from the estimated food record, the interview underestimated protein and overestimated energy, vitamin B1, and calcium, although the correlation coefficients for these were approximately 0.7 to 0.8 (de Vries et al., 2009).

She recounted a study to validate an FFQ in older Dutch men (average age of 76) in a controlled feeding trial, which provided the opportunity to compare their reported intake per the FFQ against their energy needs during the trial (de Vries et al., 2009). The FFQ was developed based on their intake according to the Dutch national food consumption survey, and the results indicated a difference in reported energy intake and energy needs of about 13 percent (the FFQ underestimated energy intake). This degree of underestimation of energy intake was similar in a study of women that compared a diet history with indirect calorimetry (Visser et al., 1995).

In nursing homes, three trained observers per ward were needed to record the daily intakes of 25 residents in fragile physical condition with cognitive decline (but not severe dementia). When compared with indirect calorimetry, the food record underestimated energy expenditure by 5 percent, and both measures reflected very low daily energy intakes.

She discussed a series of more recent (during the past decade or so) efforts to develop and improve dietary assessment tools for older adults in the Netherlands. She maintained that increasing the readability of tools is critical, such as by using drawings or icons for clarification, avoiding or at least explaining difficult words, using a different color or bolding for important words, increasing font size, shortening sentences to no more than 10 words, and adding a button for reading digitally based instruments aloud.

Next, de Vries shared an effort to develop an online screener of protein intake for hospital patients. The protein requirement is estimated based on height, weight, age, and vegetarian status, and then protein intake is assessed by questionnaire. The tool also includes information about achieving adequate intake. A similar screener for calcium was less successful, likely due to the limited number of questions asked about consumption of calcium-containing foods (Rasch et al., 2017). She mentioned another tool that used duplicate portions to assess the gluten content of diets in patients with celiac disease, which indicated that some foods contained gluten despite gluten-free claims (van der Fels-Klerx et al., 2021).

She highlighted a tool called Eetscore[5] for medical specialists to use to assess hospital patients. A short questionnaire is scored using the Dutch Healthy Diet Index,[6] and the results guide dietary advice provided to patients. Eetscore has also been adapted for use in home care via a tele-monitoring intervention to improve nutritional status (Balvers et al., 2020), which can increase patients' nutritional status. A specific application of the Eetscore to monitor micronutrient status is called NutriProfiel,[7] which combines a patient's scores with their vitamin status measured by blood biomarkers. These two metrics provide a more complete picture about vitamin sufficiency—whether insufficient status may be more likely related to dietary intake or pathophysiology—and help tailor guidance for dietary improvement and supplement intake. A study of NutriProfiel indicated that micronutrients most commonly requested for assessment are vitamin D and vitamin B12, followed by folic acid and vitamin B6, and that patients were most likely to be deficient in vitamin D.

In summary, de Vries stated that because all self-reported methodologies resulted in a relatively small underestimation of dietary intake—although most populations were comprised of healthy, educated participants—24-hour recalls or FFQs in are equally effective methods for dietary assessment in healthy older and younger people. Diet history and observation methods are burdensome, she said, and all assessment tools would benefit from further validation, particularly in lower socioeconomic populations. She also called for more information on cognitive capabilities (cognition, vision, hearing, or writing ability) to be included in evaluations of dietary assessment tools for older adults, as well as further investigation of the relationship between functionality and accurate reporting in diverse older adult populations.

ASSESSING DIETARY INTAKES AMONG OLDER ADULTS FROM DIVERSE POPULATIONS

Katherine L. Tucker, University of Massachusetts Lowell, discussed assessing dietary intakes of older adults from diverse populations. She began by reviewing challenges of dietary assessment in general, which

---

[5] https://www.wur.nl/en/show/eetscore.htm (accessed September 14, 2022).

[6] https://www.researchgate.net/publication/229434908_The_Dutch_Healthy_Diet_index_DHD-index_An_instrument_to_measure_adherence_to_the_Dutch_Guidelines_for_a_Healthy_Diet (accessed September 14, 2022).

[7] https://www.wur.nl/en/show/nutriprofiel.htm (accessed September 14, 2022).

include difficulty obtaining valid and reliable measures of nutrient intake and usual intakes over time (particularly to examine diet in relation to health outcomes), a wide diversity of populations for which assessment tools must be tailored, and the high cost and participant and/or researcher burden of doing dietary assessment well.

Tucker briefly described strengths and limitations of three traditional methods—dietary records, 24-hour dietary recalls, and FFQs. Dietary records used to be the method of choice, but they require participant literacy and cooperation, so they are often incomplete or not returned, and people tend to change their eating behavior when recording their intake.

Twenty-four-hour dietary recalls are useful and valid and have been automated and enhanced to capture intake more comprehensively, but a key limitation is that they capture only a single day. This lack of insight into day-to-day variability in intake can lead to misclassification, which she illustrated with a graph of total fat intakes of women at the 10th, 50th, and 90th percentiles over a 1-month period. Although the three percentiles are clearly separated, on a given day, the person in the 10th percentile could have been rated as the highest and the person in the 90th percentile rated quite low.

Tucker explained that the effect of that random error is that it pulls out the distribution, increasing the size of the tail by overestimating the prevalence of extreme intakes (high or low) because anyone can have an (atypical) extreme intake on a given day (Beaton, 1994). Random error also flattens the slope of the regression line, which attenuates any existing association between intake and health outcome (Beaton, 1994). True intake and more accurate distributions are more likely to be attained (particularly for foods/nutrients for which daily intake is more variable) if dietary intake is collected for a greater number of days and averaged (Basiotis et al., 1987), but the cost and burden of this approach makes it infeasible for most studies.

Tucker explained that in response to this limitation of 24-hour dietary recalls, the National Cancer Institute developed a statistical approach to adjust for day-to-day variability if at least two recalls are available for a large subset of a study population. It is useful for adjusting a population distribution and can include covariates (e.g., age, sex, ethnicity, income) but still does not accurately classify individuals (adjustments for episodically consumed foods can be applied at the population level but not on an individual level because comprehensive individual intake over the long term is not available).

The challenges of 24-hour dietary recalls have led dietary studies to rely primarily on FFQs, which provide long-term measures of usual intake with a single administration. Because FFQs cannot provide exhaustive lists of foods, they use food groupings, which can limit specificity and detail during analysis. They also make assumptions about portion sizes and recipe composition, which limit assessment of true variation and can severely underestimate intake for people with unusual intake patterns. It has been suggested that older adults with cognitive impairment cannot adequately recall intake to complete an FFQ, but with mild-to-moderate cognitive impairment and dementia, episodic memory or recall of specific details becomes reduced, whereas pattern memory (what is needed to complete an FFQ) is generally maintained (Arsenault et al., 2009; Craik et al., 1987).

Tucker highlighted the major challenges of using FFQs for diverse populations, which center on the failure of most FFQs to equally represent diets of different groups. Limited food lists may miss important ethnic foods, and cross-population differences in typical portion sizes may exist for certain foods depending on their prominence in the culture's diet. Another challenge is that differences in recipes are almost always underappreciated, even when modifications to the FFQ are attempted. These issues can produce severe bias in multicultural studies, particularly when comparing populations within a study.

Tucker elaborated on the limitations of using FFQs in diverse study populations. FFQs are designed to capture the diet of the majority group and make compromises by grouping foods and making assumptions about their relative consumption. For example, an FFQ cannot include an exhaustive list of fruits and so may have a category for "other fruits," which are assigned a weighted average and corresponding nutrient values based on population dietary intake data. However, that category may not include some or all of the fruits that certain cultures consume, which removes important variation within the study cohort. FFQs also assume standard recipes for certain foods, such as soup. The most common soup consumed in the United States is canned, so the nutrient values are based on weighted averages of popular canned varieties. But Puerto Rican populations, for example, make their own soups and consume them in larger quantities, which also contributes to bias. For example, when using well-known FFQs in certain population groups, such as Black or African American and Hispanic or Latinx individuals, bias leads to extremely low validity coefficients because important food sources of nutrients were omitted (Freeman Sullivan & Co., 1994).

Tucker discussed strategies for adapting an FFQ to a new population, based on learnings from her team's effort to modify an FFQ for a Puerto Rican adult population. The process is complicated and resource intensive, she cautioned, and starts by examining a set of representative 24-hour recalls to develop the food list (keeping in mind a country's seasonal variations for intake of certain foods). The next step is to determine the contribution weight behind the foods on the list and adjust recipes and portion sizes as needed. Tucker recounted that her team compared dietary intake information from the Hispanic Health and Nutrition Examination Survey (HHANES) against NHANES III[8] to compile its food list, rank food contributions to nutrients, modify portion sizes, and adjust recipes to reflect their contributions to nutrient intake. For example, existing FFQs assume that rice is cooked with water and a little salt, but the Puerto Rican adults eat rice in relatively large quantities and prepare it with oil. They also use tomato sauce and sofrito in many stew and bean recipes, meaning that vegetable intake would be underestimated if another recipe were used for those dishes. When the team compared both the original and modified FFQs to 24-hour recalls among Hispanic or Latino elders in Massachusetts, they observed that the original FFQ underestimated intake of all nutrients (Tucker et al., 1998).

Tucker pointed out that dietary intake differs by not only ethnicity but also region. She shared brief details about an effort to create a new FFQ for dietary assessment studies conducted in southern states in the Delta region. Many foods that were not included in well-known FFQs needed to be added to reflect the regional food sources, such as biscuits, fried catfish, cracklings, different kinds of greens, gumbo, ham hocks, sweet potato pie, and sweet tea (Tucker et al., 2005). After creating the Delta FFQ, Tucker's team was asked to produce a shortened version for the Jackson site of the Atherosclerosis Risk in Communities Study, because the study's FFQ seemed less valid in the Jackson site due to its lack of southern foods (Carithers et al., 2005).

Tucker concluded by reiterating that chronic diseases are accelerating as the world ages and urged investment in optimal dietary assessment to better understand diet's contribution to health and disease in diverse populations. She maintained that despite the desire for quick, inexpensive methods, such shortcuts do not exist when the goal is to ensure validity in intakes of different populations under study.

USING TECHNOLOGICAL APPROACHES TO RECORD DIETARY INTAKES AMONG OLDER ADULTS

Marie Kainoa Fialkowski Revilla, University of Hawai'i at Mānoa, discussed the use of technological approaches to record dietary intakes among older adults. She began by stating that this population may have physical and cognitive barriers to using technology, skeptical attitudes about its benefits, or difficulties learning how to use it (Smith, 2014). Internet usage has been rising in all age groups since 2000 and reached nearly 75 percent by 2018 among older adults (65 and older) (Faverio, 2022). For smartphones

---

[8] https://wwwn.cdc.gov/nchs/nhanes/hhanes/default.aspx (accessed September 14, 2022).

specifically, 71 percent of 65–74-year-olds and 43 percent of those 75 years and older owned one in 2021 (Gordon and Hornbrook, 2018). Technology became a key channel for connection during the COVID-19 pandemic, including among older adults (Kakulla, 2021).

Fialkowski Revilla described and image-based methods to incorporate technology into dietary assessment. A popular automated method is the Automated Self-Administered 24-hour Dietary Assessment Tool (ASA24™), a free, web-based and mobile-ready tool that can perform multiple, automatically coded, self-administered 24-hour diet recalls and/or single or multiday food records (NIH National Cancer Institute Division of Cancer Control & Population Sciences, 2022). It was used in older adults for the Interactive Diet and Activity Tracking in AARP (IDATA)[9] study, which included more than 1,100 adult AARP members aged 50–74. Participants completed six nonconsecutive ASA24s in 1 year; the method was deemed to perform as well as multiple food records and have results comparable to objective recovery biomarkers (Park et al., 2018). With respect to feasibility, 92 percent of men and 87 percent of women completed at least three ASA24s and about 75 percent overall completed at least five, a level of compliance that exceeded the levels for multiple food records or FFQs. Two-thirds or more of participants were able to complete the ASA24 on the first attempt, and more than 90 percent completed it on the second attempt; the median time to completion declined with subsequent recalls (Subar et al., 2020).

Fialkowski Revilla discussed another study that used the ASA24, the Canadian Longitudinal Study on Aging.[10] It examined the feasibility of using the ASA24-Canada-2014 version with older adults. Almost all (220) of the 232 participants completed four nonconsecutive ASA24s, although 36 percent had to do one or more by phone interview due to technological difficulties, computer literacy issues, or length (they were unable to finish independently). Results of a usability study indicated that half of participants agreed that the survey was unnecessarily complex and half said it was easy to use (Gilsing et al., 2018).

Fialkowski Revilla shared a third use of ASA24, the MoveStrong study.[11] This pilot study of 39 adults with an average age of 78 administered the ASA24-Canada by phone interview on 3 separate days. Whereas IDATA study participants took about 50 minutes to complete the ASA24 on their own, the MoveStrong study recorded average completion times of 26 minutes. The caveat to this method was that it took about six telephone calls to reach participants to complete the assessment at baseline and seven

---

[9] https://prevention.cancer.gov/research-groups/biometry/interactive-diet-and-activity (accessed September 14, 2022).

[10] https://www.clsa-elcv.ca (accessed September 14, 2022).

[11] https://the-ria.ca/project/movestrong (accessed September 14, 2022).

calls for follow-up assessments, and participants reported frustration with its specificity and repetitiousness (Wei et al., 2022).

Fialkowski Revilla discussed dietary assessment methods that rely on images. One is passive, which requires the participant to wear a device, such as a camera attached to a glasses frame, that takes images throughout the day without requiring user engagement. A contrasting approach is active, requiring the user to capture images of foods consumed throughout the day. The passive approach generates significantly more images (e.g., one image per 5 seconds or about 400,000 images/day) than the active approach (about 6–12 images/day), but most of them are not related to food and must go through a process to extract the relevant ones. An advantage of the active approach is the ability to gather information about the meal's energy, nutrients, food groups, context and location, time stamp (a marker of eating duration), and food waste.

As an example of a novel finding about temporal eating patterns and context that was enabled by using images, Fialkowski Revilla shared a study of east Asian adults (35–55 years) who completed a mobile food record with images followed by a paper food record. The number of recorded eating events was similar, but large differences existed in the times at which eating occasions were reported. The manual record showed consistent eating schedules, whereas the mobile record indicated day-to-day differences (Yonemori et al., 2022).

Fialkowski Revilla emphasized that a dietary assessment system using a mobile food record has been used to capture intake of participants across the life span, from only a few months old up to 66 years. A valuable opportunity exists to use this method along with passive methods for older adults. Research suggests that most users have compatible devices for downloading a mobile food record and are willing to do so, with the use of one's own device expected to positively influence compliance (Boushey, 2017, 312).

Fialkowski Revilla shared an incidental finding in one of her studies; grandparents were serving as surrogate reporters of infant dietary intake, which was collected via mobile food record. This finding occurs in the context of increasing U.S. prevalence of multigenerational households and provides additional evidence to suggest that older adults are willing and able to navigate the technology (Fialkowski et al., 2022). On the other hand, older adults sometimes need surrogate reporters as proxies, especially in the presence of cognitive decline. A small study of 26 older adults (65–94 years) found that when caregivers completed a 24-hour recall, the proportion of unreported foods was reduced by about 50 percent compared to when the patient did so (Pardío et al., 2016). The implication is that surrogate reporting could be a tactic for dietary assessment of older adults.

Fialkowski Revilla reiterated that smartphone ownership and Internet usage is on the rise in older adults, which presents an opportunity but must be informed by future research to assess how technology can advance dietary assessment in this population.

PANEL DISCUSSION WITH SPEAKERS

Speakers answered questions from workshop planning committee members about identifying an FFQ for a specific population and trade-offs between assessment burden and data quality.

Choosing an FFQ for Retirement Home Residents in Canada

A planning committee member noted that older adults in retirement homes where all food is provided may not have information about portion sizes or a recipe's ingredients or cooking method and may also have some degree of cognitive impairment. She asked what FFQ would be appropriate for such a population, specifically in Canada. Tucker responded that she was not aware of an FFQ that would be suitable, and she suggested developing one tailored to the target population if there are plans to examine its dietary intakes in repeated studies over time. This process begins by collecting 24-hour recalls, and comparing results to existing FFQs to evaluate whether they sufficiently capture all types of foods reported in the recalls, especially foods that might be specific to the culture or region. Boushey agreed and added that her group developed a tailored FFQ for a multiethnic cohort of native Hawaiian, Japanese American, Latino, non-Hispanic White, and African American participants. Much work was required to ensure representation of appropriate foods for these five populations, but the FFQ has worked well and complemented other assessment methods.

Trade-Offs Between Assessment Burden and Data Quality

A planning committee member recalled de Vries' comment that it took three trained observers per ward to record the daily intakes of 25 nursing home residents. She asked if it is preferable to get higher-quality data on small numbers of people than lower-quality data on large populations; de Vries acknowledged the high burden of this observational method but suggested that it is important for capturing accurate information. She noted that observers could ask kitchen staff for information about recipes and portion sizes. Another planning committee member shared her experience collecting weighted food records in a long-term care facility, which she said was "extremely labor-intensive but incredibly worthwhile" in terms of the rich data obtained. In her opinion, this level of effort is necessary for capturing intake of vulnerable populations. Tucker added that observational and weighted methods are helpful for estimating the proportion of meals that are uneaten, which she thought was important given the prevalence of poor appetites among long-term care residents. Fialkowski Revilla suggested that passive image-based methods may have utility for capturing this information in those settings.

REFERENCES

Arsenault, L. N., N. Matthan, T. M. Scott, G. Dallal, A. H. Lichtenstein, M. F. Folstein, I. Rosenberg, and K. L. Tucker. 2009. Validity of estimated dietary eicosapentaenoic acid and docosahexaenoic acid intakes determined by interviewer-administered food frequency questionnaire among older adults with mild-to-moderate cognitive impairment or dementia. *American Journal of Epidemiology* 170(1):95–103.

Bailey, R. L., D. C. Mitchell, C. K. Miller, C. D. Still, G. L. Jensen, K. L. Tucker, and H. Smiciklas-Wright. 2007. A dietary screening questionnaire identifies dietary patterns in older adults. *Journal of Nutrition* 137(2):421–426.

Balvers, M., M. De Rijk, A. Slotegraaf, J. K. Gunnewiek, and J. De Vries. 2020. Development and implementation of online tools for personalized dietary advice at home or in a clinical setting: Eetscore and NutriProfiel. *Proceedings of the Nutrition Society* 79(OCE2):E526.

Basiotis, P. P., S. O. Welsh, F. J. Cronin, J. L. Kelsay, and W. Mertz. 1987. Number of days of food intake records required to estimate individual and group nutrient intakes with defined confidence. *Journal of Nutrition* 117(9):1638–1641.

Beaton, G. H. 1994. Approaches to analysis of dietary data: Relationship between planned analyses and choice of methodology. *American Journal of Clinical Nutrition* 59(1 Suppl):253S–261S.

Boushey, C. J., M. Spoden, E. J. Delp, F. Zhu, M. Bosch, Z. Ahmad, Y. B. Shvetsov, J. P. DeLany, and D. A. Kerr. 2017. Reported energy intake accuracy compared to doubly labeled water and usability of the mobile food record among community dwelling adults. *Nutrients* 9(3):312.

Carithers, T., P. M. Dubbert, E. Crook, B. Davy, S. B. Wyatt, M. L. Bogle, H. A. Taylor, Jr., and K. L. Tucker. 2005. Dietary assessment in African Americans: Methods used in the Jackson Heart Study. *Ethnicity and Disease* 15(4 Suppl 6):S6-49–55.

Craik, F. I. M., M. Byrd, and J. M. Swanson. 1987. Patterns of memory loss in three elderly samples. *Psychology and Aging* 2(1):79–86.

de Vries, J. H., L. C. de Groot, and W. A. van Staveren. 2009. Dietary assessment in elderly people: Experiences gained from studies in the Netherlands. *European Journal of Clinical Nutrition* 63(Suppl 1):S69–S74.

Faverio, M. 2022. *Share of those 65 and older who are tech users has grown in the past decade.* Washington, DC: Pew Research Center.

Fialkowski, M. K., J. Kai, C. Young, G. Langfelder, J. Ng-Osorio, Z. Shao, F. Zhu, D. A. Kerr, and C. J. Boushey. 2022. An active image-based mobile food record is feasible for capturing eating occasions among infants ages 3–12 months old in Hawai'i. *Nutrients* 14(5).

Ford, D. W., T. J. Hartman, C. Still, C. Wood, D. Mitchell, P. Y. Hsiao, R. Bailey, H. Smiciklas-Wright, D. L. Coffman, and G. L. Jensen. 2014. Diet-related practices and BMI are associated with diet quality in older adults. *Public Health Nutrition* 17(7):1565–1569.

Freeman Sullivan and Co. 1994. *WIC Dietary Assessment Validation Study.* Alexandria, VA: U.S. Department of Agriculture Food and Nutrition Service.

Gilsing, A., A. J. Mayhew, H. Payette, B. Shatenstein, S. I. Kirkpatrick, K. Amog, C. Wolfson, S. Kirkland, L. E. Griffith, and P. Raina. 2018. Validity and reliability of a short diet questionnaire to estimate dietary intake in older adults in a subsample of the Canadian Longitudinal Study on Aging. *Nutrients* 10(10).

Gordon, N. P., and M. C. Hornbrook. 2018. Older adults' readiness to engage with ehealth patient education and self-care resources: A cross-sectional survey. *BMC Health Services Research* 18(1):220.

Greene, G. W., I. Lofgren, C. Paulin, M. L. Greaney, and P. G. Clark. 2018. Differences in psychosocial and behavioral variables by dietary screening tool risk category in older adults. *Journal of the Academy of Nutrition and Dietetics* 118(1):110–117.

Jacka, F. N., A. O'Neil, R. Opie, C. Itsiopoulos, S. Cotton, M. Mohebbi, D. Castle, S. Dash, C. Mihalopoulos, M. L. Chatterton, L. Brazionis, O. M. Dean, A. M. Hodge, and M. Berk. 2017. A randomised controlled trial of dietary improvement for adults with major depression (the "SMILES" trial). *BMC Medicine* 15(1):23.

Johnson, E. J., R. Vishwanathan, M. A. Johnson, D. B. Hausman, A. Davey, T. M. Scott, R. C. Green, L. S. Miller, M. Gearing, J. Woodard, P. T. Nelson, H. Y. Chung, W. Schalch, J. Wittwer, and L. W. Poon. 2013. Relationship between serum and brain carotenoids, alpha-tocopherol, and retinol concentrations and cognitive performance in the oldest old from the Georgia Centenarian Study. *Journal of Aging Research* 951786.

Johnson, M. A., A. Davey, S. Park, D. B. Hausman, L. W. Poon, and The Georgia Centenarian Study. 2008. Age, race and season predict vitamin D status in African American and White octogenarians and centenarians. *Journal of Nutrition, Health & Aging* 12(10):690–695.

Johnson, M. A., D. B. Hausman, A. Davey, L. W. Poon, R. H. Allen, S. P. Stabler, and The Georgia Centenarian Study. 2010. Vitamin B12 deficiency in African American and White octogenarians and centenarians in Georgia. *Journal of Nutrition, Health & Aging* 14(5):339–345.

Kakulla, B. April 2021. *2021 tech trends and the 50-plus: Top 10 biggest trends.* Washington, DC: AARP Research.

Kwak, C. S., M. S. Lee, S. I. Oh, and S. C. Park. 2010. Discovery of novel sources of vitamin B(12) in traditional Korean foods from nutritional surveys of centenarians. *Current Gerontology and Geriatrics Research* 374897.

Looker, A. C., B. Dawson-Hughes, M. S. Calvo, E. W. Gunter, and N. R. Sahyoun. 2002. Serum 25-hydroxyvitamin D status of adolescents and adults in two seasonal subpopulations from NHANES III. *Bone* 30(5):771–777.

Mitchell, D. C., K. L. Tucker, J. Maras, F. R. Lawrence, H. Smiciklas-Wright, G. L. Jensen, C. D. Still, and T. J. Hartman. 2012. Relative validity of the Geisinger Rural Aging Study food frequency questionnaire. *Journal of Nutrition, Health & Aging* 16(7):667–672.

Mohn, E., R. Vishwanathan, W. Schalch, A. Lichtenstein, N. Matthan, and L. Poon. 2013. *The relationship of lutein and DHA in age-related cognitive function.* Paper presented at the Experimental Biology Conference, Boston, MA.

NIH National Cancer Institute Division of Cancer Control & Population Sciences. 2022. *Automated Self-Administered 24-hour (ASA24) Dietary Assessment Tool.* https://epi.grants.cancer.gov/asa24/ (accessed September 14, 2022).

Pardío, J., P. Arroyo, A. Loría, S. Torres-Castro, M. Agudelo-Botero, B. L. Jiménez Herrera, and A. T. Serrano Miranda. 2016. Accuracy of 24-hr food-registry method in elderly subjects: Role of a surrogate respondent. *Journal of Aging Research Clinical Practice* 5(4):217–219.

Park, Y., K. W. Dodd, V. Kipnis, F. E. Thompson, N. Potischman, D. A. Schoeller, D. J. Baer, D. Midthune, R. P. Troiano, H. Bowles, and A. F. Subar. 2018. Comparison of self-reported dietary intakes from the automated self-administered 24-h recall, 4-D food records, and food-frequency questionnaires against recovery biomarkers. *American Journal of Clinical Nutrition* 107(1):80–93.

Passeri, G., G. Pini, L. Troiano, R. Vescovini, P. Sansoni, M. Passeri, P. Gueresi, R. Delsignore, M. Pedrazzoni, and C. Franceschi. 2003. Low vitamin D status, high bone turnover, and bone fractures in centenarians. *International Journal of Clinical Endocrinology and Metabolism* 88(11):5109–5115.

Poon, L. W., M. Jazwinski, R. C. Green, J. L. Woodard, P. Martin, W. L. Rodgers, M. A. Johnson, D. Hausman, J. Arnold, A. Davey, M. A. Batzer, W. R. Markesbery, M. Gearing, I. C. Siegler, S. Reynolds, and J. Dai. 2007. Methodological considerations in studying centenarians: Lessons learned from the Georgia Centenarian Studies. *Annual Review of Gerontology and Geriatrics* 27(1):231–264.

Rasch, L. A., M. A. de van der Schueren, L. H. van Tuyl, I. E. Bultink, J. H. de Vries, and W. F. Lems. 2017. Content validity of a short calcium intake list to estimate daily dietary calcium intake of patients with osteoporosis. *Calcified Tissue International* 100(3):271–277.

Shaw, K., M. Gearing, A. Davey, M. Burgess, L. W. Poon, P. Martin, and R. C. Green. 2012. Successful recruitment of centenarians for post-mortem brain donation: Results from the Georgia Centenarian Study. *Journal of Biosciences and Medicines* 2(1).

Smith, A. 2014. *Older adults and technology use.* Washington, DC: Pew Research Center.

Statista. 2022. Number of people aged 100 and older (centenarians) worldwide from 2010 to 2100 (in 1,000s). Hamberg, Germany: Statista.

Subar, A. F., N. Potischman, K. W. Dodd, F. E. Thompson, D. J. Baer, D. A. Schoeller, D. Midthune, V. Kipnis, S. I. Kirkpatrick, B. Mittl, T. P. Zimmerman, D. Douglass, H. R. Bowles, and Y. Park. 2020. Performance and feasibility of recalls completed using the Automated Self-Administered 24-hour Dietary Assessment Tool in relation to other self-report tools and biomarkers in the Interactive Diet and Activity Tracking in AARP (IDATA) study. *Journal of the Academy of Nutrition and Dietetics* 120(11):1805–1820.

Tucker, K. L., L. A. Bianchi, J. Maras, and O. I. Bermudez. 1998. Adaptation of a food frequency questionnaire to assess diets of Puerto Rican and non-Hispanic adults. *American Journal of Epidemiology* 148(5):507–518.

Tucker, K. L., J. Maras, C. Champagne, C. Connell, S. Goolsby, J. Weber, S. Zaghloul, T. Carithers, and M. L. Bogle. 2005. A regional food-frequency questionnaire for the U.S. Mississippi Delta. *Public Health Nutrition* 8(1):87–96.

van der Fels-Klerx, H. J., N. G. E. Smits, M. Bremer, J. M. Schultink, M. M. Nijkamp, J. J. M. Castenmiller, and J. H. M. de Vries. 2021. Detection of gluten in duplicate portions to determine gluten intake of coeliac disease patients on a gluten-free diet. *British Journal of Nutrition* 125(9):1051–1057.

Ventura Marra, M., S. V. Thuppal, E. J. Johnson, and R. L. Bailey. 2018. Validation of a dietary screening tool in a middle-aged Appalachian population. *Nutrients* 10(3).

Visser, M., L. C. De Groot, P. Deurenberg, and W. A. Van Staveren. 1995. Validation of dietary history method in a group of elderly women using measurements of total energy expenditure. *British Journal of Nutrition* 74(6):775–785.

Wei, C., J. B. Wagler, I. B. Rodrigues, L. Giangregorio, H. Keller, L. Thabane, and M. Mourtzakis. 2022. Telephone administration of the automated self-administered 24-hour dietary assessment in older adults: Lessons learned. *Canadian Journal of Dietetic Practice and Research* 83(1):30–34.

Willett, W. 2013. *Nutritional epidemiology.* U.S.: Oxford University Press.

Yonemori, K. M., L. Zuccarelli, L. Le Marchand, F. M. Zhu, D. Kerr, and C. J. Boushey. 2022. Temporal patterns of eating by mode of data collection from the baseline dietary intakes of participants in the Healthy Diet and Lifestyle Study. *Journal of Food Composition and Analysis* 107:104296.

4

Nutritional Screening of Older Adults

BOX 4-1
HIGHLIGHTS[a]

- Nutrition screening is a critical first step to identify which individuals warrant comprehensive nutrition assessment. Screening identifies risk for a specific outcome related to nutritional status and is less comprehensive and resource intensive than nutrition assessment, which is an in-depth, specific, detailed evaluation to clarify etiology, severity, and appropriate intervention and outcome monitoring. (Jensen)
- This workshop focused on screening for risk of protein-energy malnutrition or malnutrition, henceforth referred to as "malnutrition." This condition occurs when intake or uptake of energy and/or protein is lower than that required by the body for weight maintenance and physiological functioning. The delivery of sufficient energy and/or protein can be compromised by inadequate consumption, nutrient assimilation disorders, and higher energy and/or protein requirements influenced by the disease process, including inflammatory conditions within the body. (Jensen)
- According to the European Malnutrition in the Elderly (MaNuEL) project, close to 23 percent of European older adults are at high risk and nearly 50 percent are at some risk for malnutrition. Similar prevalence is observed in the United States and Canada. Therefore, malnutrition screening of older adults is highly important. (van der Schueren)
- Since the 1990s, key milestones in the evolution of malnutrition screening include developing tools specifically designed for this purpose, most notably the Nutrition Screening Initiative (incorporating the Determine Your Health Checklist and Level I and II screens) and the Mini Nutritional Assessment. (Jensen)

- During the past several decades, many more malnutrition screening tools have been developed to serve one of three purposes: identifying risk of malnutrition, predicting outcomes related to nutritional status, or predicting response to nutritional support. The choice of tool depends on the screening's goal and setting, but many tools are neither used for their intended objectives nor applied in the population for which they were developed and validated. Furthermore, a number of screening tools have been used to evaluate nutritional status, and several nutrition assessment tools have been used to screen for malnutrition, thus blurring the line between screening and assessment. (van der Schueren)
- Food insecurity and low income are associated with poor nutrient intake and dietary quality, higher prevalence of overweight and obesity, and higher prevalence of chronic diseases. The nutrition risks associated with older age are compounded by low income and food insecurity, such that increased nutrition needs may be harder to achieve. An analysis of these topics found that about 40 percent of U.S. adults who are aged ≥60 with low incomes had food insecurity and about 60 percent used dietary supplements. Dietary quality and nutrient intake from food alone were very poor among older adults with low incomes, but nutrient intake was improved among supplement users. However, total dietary quality was not significantly different between supplement users and nonusers. (Eicher-Miller)
- Little is known about the nutritional challenges of older adults of advanced age (i.e., ≥80). Recent research in Denmark that examined this topic found that protein malnutrition is prevalent but that in primary prevention settings, this status may not be detectable based on unintentional weight loss, low BMI, or other typical malnutrition indicators. Furthermore, weight loss, dental status, dysphagia, and high BMI were independently associated with physical pre-frail or frail status among older adults of advanced age, and the presence of two or more factors, among a broader list of nutritional risk factors, was associated with more than a twofold increased risk for pre-frail/frail status. (Buhl)

---

[a]This list is the rapporteurs' summary of points made by the individual speakers identified, and the statements have not been endorsed or verified by the National Academies of Sciences, Engineering, and Medicine. They are not intended to reflect a consensus among workshop participants.

The third workshop, held April 29, 2022, featured four presentations about screening for malnutrition in older adults, followed by a panel discussion with the speakers. Presentation topics included experiences with screening for malnutrition in the United States and internationally and how food insecurity can negatively affect nutritional status. Gordon Jensen, University of Vermont, and Clare Corish, University College Dublin, moderated the workshop.

A U.S. EXPERIENCE WITH SCREENING FOR MALNUTRITION: THE NUTRITION SCREENING INITIATIVE TO 2022

Jensen provided a brief historical overview of screening for deteriorating nutritional status and/or malnutrition in older U.S. adults from the 1990s development and implementation of the Nutrition Screening Initiative[1] to the present day. The risk factors for a deterioration in nutritional status are many, including poor food intake, food insecurity, poverty, isolation, functional limitations, disease, polypharmacy, poor dentition, alcohol and substance use, depression, and dementia. Screening approaches have incorporated these risk factors; he clarified the clear differences between screening for risk of malnutrition and assessment of the condition. Nutrition screening identifies risk for a specific outcome related to nutritional status, such as functional decline, health care resource use, or malnutrition, whereas nutrition assessment is an in-depth, specific, detailed evaluation to clarify etiology, severity, and appropriate intervention and the intervention outcomes that require monitoring thereafter. He emphasized that screening is less comprehensive and thus requires fewer resources than assessment, which is a more robust evaluation that is more time consuming and takes higher levels of training and skills.

Jensen recounted details of the Nutrition Screening Initiative, which was introduced in the late 1990s through a collaboration of the American Academy of Family Physicians, American Dietetic Association, and National Council on Aging as the first major initiative to promote screening of nutritional status in older adults. The most widely promoted aspect was the Determine Your Nutritional Health checklist, which captured nine risk factors and enabled older adults to tally their self-reported nutritional health status and determine their standing of low, moderate, or high risk (Figure 4-1).

The checklist, meant as a tool to raise public and self-awareness, ended up being used in many applications (e.g., full nutrition assessments in hospitals) for which it was neither intended nor validated, and validation highlighted some limitations. He referenced one example, a 1993 study that examined its application in a Medicare beneficiary population and found that its sensitivity was poor for identifying low nutrient ingestion or perceived poor health (Posner et al., 1993). A few years later, another study reported that some checklist items were significantly associated with mortality. Overall consideration of study results suggested that the checklist might best serve as an awareness and educational tool for older adults and their caregivers (Sahyoun et al., 1997).

---

[1] https://www.sciencedirect.com/topics/medicine-and-dentistry/nutrition-screening#:~: text=Nutrition%20Screening%20Initiative%20(NSI)&text=It%20was%20created%20as%20 part,in%20different%20settings%20%5B17%5D (accessed September 14, 2022).

The Warning Signs of poor nutritional health are often overlooked. Use this checklist to find out if you or someone you know is at nutritional risk.

Read the statements below. Circle the number in the yes column for those that apply to you or someone you know. For each yes answer, score the number in the box. Total your nutritional score.

DETERMINE YOUR NUTRITIONAL HEALTH

	YES
I have an illness or condition that made me change the kind and/or amount of food I eat.	2
I eat fewer than 2 meals per day.	3
I eat few fruits or vegetables, or milk products.	2
I have 3 or more drinks of beer, liquor or wine almost every day.	2
I have tooth or mouth problems that make it hard for me to eat.	2
I don't always have enough money to buy the food I need.	4
I eat alone most of the time.	1
I take 3 or more different prescribed or over-the-counter drugs a day.	1
Without wanting to, I have lost or gained 10 pounds in the last 6 months.	2
I am not always physically able to shop, cook and/or feed myself.	2
TOTAL	

Total Your Nutritional Score. If it's —

0-2 Good! Recheck your nutritional score in 6 months.

3-5 You are at moderate nutritional risk. See what can be done to improve your eating habits and lifestyle. Your office on aging, senior nutrition program, senior citizens center or health department can help. Recheck your nutritional score in 3 months.

6 or more You are at high nutritional risk. Bring this checklist the next time you see your doctor, dietitian or other qualified health or social service professional. Talk with them about any problems you may have. Ask for help to improve your nutritional health.

These materials developed and distributed by the Nutrition Screening Initiative, a project of the

AMERICAN ACADEMY of FAMILY PHYSICIANS

THE AMERICAN DIETETIC ASSOCIATION

NATIONAL COUNCIL ON THE AGING, INC.

produced in part through a grant from Ross Products Division, Abbott Laboratories.

Remember that warning signs suggest risk, but do not represent diagnosis of any condition. Turn the page to learn more about the Warning Signs of poor nutritional health.

The Nutrition Screening Initiative • 1010 Wisconsin Avenue, NW • Suite 800 • Washington, DC 20007

The Nutrition Checklist is based on the Warning Signs described below. Use the word DETERMINE to remind you of the Warning Signs.

DISEASE
Any disease, illness or chronic condition which causes you to change the way you eat, or makes it hard for you to eat, puts your nutritional health at risk. Four out of five adults have chronic diseases that are affected by diet. Confusion or memory loss that keeps getting worse is estimated to affect one out of five or more of older adults. This can make it hard to remember what, when or if you've eaten. Feeling sad or depressed, which happens to about one in eight older adults, can cause big changes in appetite, digestion, energy level, weight and well-being.

EATING POORLY
Eating too little and eating too much both lead to poor health. Eating the same foods day after day or not eating fruit, vegetables, and milk products daily will also cause poor nutritional health. One in five adults skip meals daily. Only 13% of adults eat the minimum amount of fruit and vegetables needed. One in four older adults drink too much alcohol. Many health problems become worse if you drink more than one or two alcoholic beverages per day.

TOOTH LOSS/ MOUTH PAIN
A healthy mouth, teeth and gums are needed to eat. Missing, loose or rotten teeth or dentures which don't fit well or cause mouth sores make it hard to eat.

ECONOMIC HARDSHIP
As many as 40% of older Americans have incomes of less than $6,000 per year. Having less—or choosing to spend less—than $25-30 per week for food makes it very hard to get the foods you need to stay healthy.

REDUCED SOCIAL CONTACT
One-third of all older people live alone. Being with people every day has a positive effect on morale, well-being and eating.

MULTIPLE MEDICINES
Many older Americans must take medicines for health problems. Almost half of older Americans take multiple medicines daily. Growing old may change the way we respond to drugs. The more medicines you take, the greater the chance for side effects such as increased or decreased appetite, change in taste, constipation, weakness, drowsiness, diarrhea, nausea, and others. Vitamins or minerals when taken in large doses act like drugs and can cause harm. Alert your doctor to everything you take.

INVOLUNTARY WEIGHT LOSS/GAIN
Losing or gaining a lot of weight when you are not trying to do so is an important warning sign that must not be ignored. Being overweight or underweight also increases your chance of poor health.

NEEDS ASSISTANCE IN SELF CARE
Although most older people are able to eat, one of every five have trouble walking, shopping, buying and cooking food, especially as they get older.

ELDER YEARS ABOVE AGE 80
Most older people lead full and productive lives. But as age increases, risk of frailty and health problems increase. Checking your nutritional health regularly makes good sense.

The Nutrition Screening Initiative • 1010 Wisconsin Avenue, NW • Suite 800 • Washington, DC 20007
The Nutrition Screening Initiative is funded in part by a grant from Ross Laboratories, a Division of Abbott Laboratories.

FIGURE 4-1 Determine Your Nutritional Health checklist from the Nutrition Screening Initiative.
SOURCE: Presented by Gordon Jensen on April 29, 2022.

The Nutrition Screening Initiative released two further tools, a Level I screen that he described as "a step toward assessment" and a Level II screen that was a full-fledged nutrition assessment tool. The Level II screen was intended for use by health care professionals in acute, chronic, and long-term care settings. Jensen explained that it combined the Level 1 screen with more formal assessment variables, which included physical signs and symptoms of deficiency, laboratory testing, and evaluation of cognitive and emotional status using questions from the Mini-Mental State Exam (MMSE) and questions on depression.

According to Jensen, neither tool had widespread application, but he referenced the Level II screen's use in the Geisinger Rural Aging Study (GRAS) (see Chapter 3) in rural central Pennsylvania. It was administered during enrollment clinic visits in the late 1990s, during which participants completed self-report questions with nurse-measured height and weight. More than 21,600 people 65 years and older enrolled during 1994–1999, and they have received follow-up questionnaires by mail every 3–4 years. The researchers also received data in the form of annual downloads of deidentified electronic health record data from the Geisinger Healthcare System. Over the past 25 years, they have continued to monitor mortality and health outcomes in relation to nutrition risk status.

Jensen referred to Mitchell's presentation about GRAS (see Chapter 3) in highlighting the comprehensive evaluations conducted with representative subsets of the study cohort. He reiterated what she shared in terms of key findings from the two-plus decades of GRAS research: high prevalence of poor-quality diets, obesity, and poor health; association of obesity with comorbidity and functional decline; and association of low diet quality with lower body mass index (BMI) and increased mortality (Jensen et al., 1997). The study has 177 confirmed centenarians, and its researchers are examining nutrition risk, quality of life, and health outcomes as predictors of living to 100.

Jensen shared results from an evaluation of malnutrition screening focused on older adults (the Mini Nutrional Assessment [MNA][2]) that included BMI, calf circumference, weight loss, living environment, mobility, mental status, medications, pressure wounds, dietary habits, self-perceived health, and nutrition. Discriminate analysis comparing the MNA to a comprehensive gold standard of clinical, anthropometric, laboratory, and dietary measures indicated its high levels of sensitivity (96 percent), specificity (98 percent), and predictive value (97 percent) (Vellas et al., 1999). Jensen highlighted that the authors of that work published a paper in 2021 summarizing their 25 years with the MNA, which has included develop-

[2] https://www.mna-elderly.com/sites/default/files/2021-10/mna-mini-english.pdf (accessed September 14, 2022).

ing full, short-form, and self-reported MNAs, and the completion of 2,000 reported studies using the MNA (Guigoz and Vellas, 2021).

Jensen described a more recent (Silva et al., 2020) systematic review that examined malnutrition risk screening tools for older adults with COVID-19. It included studies that examined a variety of different screening and assessment tools. The authors noted that most of the instruments had high sensitivity for identifying risk of malnutrition, but none stood out as the best (Silva et al., 2020). The implication of this finding is that it may be about developing tools for not only specific cohorts but possibly even specific types of diseases and disorders, acknowledging that developing and validating a screening tool is a considerable undertaking.

AN INTERNATIONAL EXPERIENCE WITH SCREENING FOR MALNUTRITION

Marian de van der Schueren, Han University, described a European experience with screening older adults for malnutrition. She began with a definition of the screening: a quick and easy procedure using a valid tool, designed to identify those who are malnourished or at risk of malnutrition and may benefit from nutritional intervention from a registered dietitian or clinician with nutrition training (Kondrup et al., 2003). She echoed Jensen's delineation between screening and assessment and added that screening is only the first step in the nutritional management of older adults.

She observed that a plethora of screening tools have been developed during the past 10–20 years, many of which have been designed and validated for older adults. She explained that most tools are developed to serve one of three purposes: to identify risk of malnutrition, predict outcomes related to nutritional status, or predict response to nutritional support. In the Netherlands, the Short Nutritional Assessment Questionnaire (SNAQ)[3] is often used to identify risk of malnutrition, and other tools for this purpose include the Nutritional Risk Screening (NRS),[4] MNA,[5] Nutritional Risk Index (NRI),[6] and Malnutrition Universal Screening Tool (MUST).[7] She explained that although each tool was developed and validated specifically for one of the three listed purposes, the reality is that tools intended for malnutrition are also used for the other two purposes and vice versa.

---

[3] https://www.fightmalnutrition.eu/toolkits/summary-screening-tools (accessed September 14, 2022).

[4] https://www.ncbi.nlm.nih.gov/pmc/articles/PMC6679209 (accessed September 14, 2022).

[5] https://www.mna-elderly.com/sites/default/files/2021-10/mna-mini-english.pdf (accessed September 14, 2022).

[6] https://www.sciencedirect.com/science/article/pii/B9780128179901000469 (accessed September 14, 2022).

[7] https://www.bapen.org.uk/pdfs/must/must_full.pdf (accessed September 14, 2022).

Similarly, some tools developed and validated for older adults (e.g., the MNA and the Geriatric Nutrition Risk Index [GNRI]) are used for younger adults and vice versa.

She discussed her experience as a collaborator on the European Malnutrition in the Elderly project (MaNuEL).[8] She described three of the project studies: a review of the validity of malnutrition screening tools used in older adults, development of a scoring system to rate these tools in older adults, and a systematic review of malnutrition risk among older adults in Europe. All three focused on protein-energy malnutrition specifically in older adults.

The review of the validity of malnutrition screening tools examined 48 tools that had been applied in studies with older adults and found that 34 were validated for use in one of four settings: community, rehabilitation, residential care institutions, or hospitals (Power et al., 2018). Some validated tools had been used in only one study and others in as many as nine studies. The tool(s) with greatest evidence of validity for each setting was the SCREEN II instrument (community), the Nutritional Form for the Elderly (NUFFE) (rehabilitation), SNAQ (residential care institutions), and MUST and the Malnutrition Screening Tool (MST; hospitals).

She then discussed the scoring system to rate malnutrition screening tools, which sought to identify which tools rated most highly for being quick, simple, and valid in the same four settings examined in the first MaNuEL study (Power et al., 2019). The research team examined the 48 tools identified in that review and observed that each tool consisted of different items: biochemical measures, anthropometric measures, subjective measures of physical functioning (e.g., difficulty with mobility), social function (e.g., financial situation, access to food), cognitive function (e.g., mental distress/illness, living alone, loss of a partner, dementia), or a combination of these items.

The team developed a rating system underpinned by scientific literature and expert consensus, de van der Schueren said, and scored the 48 tools for their validation, scientific evidence for the included parameters in assessing risk of malnutrition in older adults, and practicability. She explained that each tool was evaluated based on whether it had been validated for use in older adults, the type of validity assessed (construct, criterion, or predictive), the gold standard against which it had been validated, the results (e.g., sensitivity and specificity), and the number of validation studies performed. The team identified 54 parameters with varying levels of evidence. For example, some parameters were deemed not suitable for use (e.g., serum albumin) compared to others (e.g., questions about recent weight loss and appetite). In terms of practicability, the tools were rated based on

---

[8] https://www.healthydietforhealthylife.eu/index.php/news/232-manuel-the-knowledge-hub-on-malnutrition-in-the-elderly (accessed September 14, 2022).

the time required, associated costs, availability in multiple languages, and how widely the tool could be used (i.e., a tool that required staff trained in nutrition scored less well than one that could be used by all staff with minimal training). The tools with the highest scores for each setting were the Determine Your Health Checklist (community), NUFFE (rehabilitation), SNAQ (residential care), and MNA and MST (hospital).

Moving onto the third study, de van der Schueren explained that the systematic review of malnutrition risk in older adults in Europe was based on studies that had used the 22 best-rated malnutrition screening tools (according to the prior MaNuEL studies) validated for use in older adults (Leij-Halfwerk et al., 2019). The research team identified 223 study populations that were examined across the four settings (138 populations were hospital inpatients) comprising more than 500,000 hospital inpatients, almost 3,000 from rehabilitation settings, more than 22,000 from residential care settings, and more than 30,000 from community settings.

The pooled prevalence rates of malnutrition risk in European older adults, combined for health care settings, countries, and malnutrition screening tools, were 22.6 percent for high risk and 48.4 percent for moderate plus high risk (Leij-Halfwerk, 2019, p. 24). She described these results as an important public health consideration, adding that when examined by individual country, the pooled prevalence rates for moderate plus high malnutrition risk ranged from 41 percent in Spain to 67 percent in Finland.

The team also examined malnutrition risk by four of the screening tools (combined for all countries and health care settings) for which adequate power was available, finding that different prevalence rates for both high and moderate plus high malnutrition resulted for each tool (Leij-Halfwerk, 2019, p. 24). The greatest prevalence of high (40.6 percent) and moderate plus high (62.3 percent) risk came from the NRS-2002, for example, and the lowest (19.0 and 39.7 percent, respectively) from the GNRI. When malnutrition risk was examined by health care setting, the highest risk was from hospital settings (28.0 percent for high risk and 53.0 percent for moderate plus high risk) and the lowest from community settings (8.5 and 32.7 percent, respectively).

The key results of the meta-analysis were that close to 23 out of 100 European older adults are at high risk for malnutrition and nearly 50 percent are at any risk for malnutrition. Older age (>80 years) and female gender were associated with higher risk, and differences were observed by health care setting, country, and tool. The results led the researchers to conclude that standardized use of one preferred screening tool per health care setting is strongly recommended.

The three MaNuEL studies occurred just before the 2019 launch of the Global Leadership Initiative in Malnutrition (GLIM), de van der Schueren said, which aims to develop a consensus-based, standardized framework for malnutrition risk screening and diagnosis in adults across settings and countries (Cederholm et al., 2019; Jensen et al., 2019). GLIM was the first globally accepted approach to malnutrition diagnosis despite broad use of several select malnutrition indicators across continents and countries. In addition, in many regions of the world, access to skilled nutrition professionals and resources is limited, making it necessary to develop and disseminate a simplified approach. The GLIM framework is a global consensus project to help address these issues. The key steps in the framework are to conduct malnutrition risk screening using validated tools, perform a diagnostic assessment consisting of phenotypic and etiologic criteria, and determine if the patient meets criteria for a malnutrition diagnosis. She noted that GLIM continues to be refined, highlighting that one challenge in this process is that different tools have different goals (are screening for different things).

To illustrate the different goals of various tools, de van der Schueren described her team's effort to screen 200 community-dwelling older adults (without known specific nutritional problems) for malnutrition risk (Borkent et al., 2020). The team used the SNAQ65+ (a version of the questionnaire for adults ≥65 years of age) and the Seniors in the Community: Risk Evaluation for Eating and Nutrition (SCREEN II). The SNAQ65+ screens for malnutrition (characterized by weight loss, impaired muscle mass, and functional difficulties), whereas the SCREEN II screens for risk factors associated with the development of malnutrition. The prevalence of malnutrition was close to 14 percent according to SNAQ65+ and 69 percent according to SCREEN II. It is likely that these differences would influence malnutrition prevalence using GLIM or other approaches to diagnosis.

She shared several take-home messages about malnutrition screening. First, it is important for older adults, given that malnutrition appears to affect up to half of this population, and it is critical to use tools validated for older adults compared to those validated for the general adult population. The choice of tool depends on the goal of screening, such as the example illustrating the differences between the SNAQ and SCREEN II, and also on the setting of the screening. She urged implementation of a system to screen for malnutrition in all health care settings. In the Netherlands, for example, malnutrition risk screening is mandatory in everyone admitted to the hospital; she thinks that has helped advance the nutritional care of older adults.

SCREENING FOR FOOD INSECURITY

Heather Eicher-Miller, Purdue University, discussed food insecurity in older adults, its relationship to poverty, and the association between poor nutrient intake and dietary quality and living in a low-income, food insecure situation. She stated that the prevalence of low incomes among U.S. adults aged 65 and older is about 9 percent (U.S. Census Bureau, 2021), and having low income presents both nutrition and health risks. This is because a limited income constrains food selection to more economical options that are then subject to other decision-making considerations, such as time and equipment available for food preparation, cooking interest and skills, taste preferences, and cultural considerations.

Low income is defined by federal poverty guidelines, which are based on official poverty thresholds that vary by family size and composition and are updated annually (Figure 4-2). If a family's total income is less than the family threshold, it is considered to be "in poverty." This is the only population segment officially defined by income level, and the poverty threshold includes the criterion that one-third or more of a household's expenses after taxes is needed to purchase food (based on the cost of USDA's thrifty food plan).

Food insecurity, defined as household uncertainty of having or being able to acquire enough food to meet all members' needs because of insufficient money, is most prevalent among households with incomes near or below the poverty line (Marshall, 2010). Eicher-Miller pointed out that

Persons in family/household	Poverty guideline
1	$12,880
2	$17,420
3	$21,960
4	$26,500
5	$31,040
6	$35,580
7	$40,120
8	$44,660
For families/households with more than 8 persons, add $4,540 for each additional person.	

FIGURE 4-2 2021 poverty guidelines for the 48 contiguous states and the District of Columbia.
SOURCE: Presented by Heather Eicher-Miller on April 29, 2022 (ASPE, 2021).

despite some degree of subjectivity in self-reporting sufficient food, this is highly associated with income. Food security can be quantified using the U.S. Household Food Security Survey, an 18-item, self-report questionnaire that assesses concerns about having enough food and whether a household is eating differently because of not having enough resources for food. The results classify households as having food security, low food security (i.e., self-reported reduced dietary quality), or very low food security (i.e., self-reported reduced amount of food consumed). In 2020, 89.5 percent of households were classified as food secure, 6.6 percent as low food secure, and 3.9 percent as very low food secure (Coleman-Jensen et al., 2021). A 2014 survey examined food insecurity among older adults (ages 65–84) specifically, finding that 20 percent of those with a poverty-income ratio of less than three were food insecure (Miller et al., 2020). That ratio is defined as "the ratio of income to the poverty threshold set by the U.S. Census Bureau (adjusted for inflation and family size)" (Miller et al., 2020).

Eicher-Miller discussed the association of poor health and diet with living in a low-income, food insecure situation. Populations that experience food insecurity and low income have poorer nutrient intakes and dietary quality and higher prevalence of overweight, obesity, and chronic diseases, such as diabetes, heart disease, and cancer, compared to populations that are food secure (Bailey et al., 2017; Cowan et al., 2019; Hiza et al., 2013; Holben and Pheley, 2006; Pan et al., 2012; Seligman et al., 2010). A research gap exists in that more studies have examined different or broader age groups than older adults with low incomes and/or food insecurity. The nutrition risks associated with older age (i.e., reduced metabolic rate, decreased bodily functions and mobility, and reduced digestion and absorption of nutrients) are compounded by low income and food insecurity, such that their increased nutrition needs may be harder to achieve. For example, older adults may have reduced access to transportation to obtain food, reduced physical mobility for preparing food, fewer resources for food, and lower access to health care and other wellness resources (Barbagallo et al., 2009; Luhrmann et al., 2009; Russell, 2001; Veldurthy et al., 2016; Volpi et al., 2004).

Eicher-Miller pointed out that nutrients that support healthy aging and that might be of greater need for older adults (protein, calcium, magnesium, zinc, vitamins A, B6, B12, C, D, E and folate) are the same (save vitamin B12) as the list of those that have lower intake in low- versus high-income groups and food-secure versus food-insecure groups (Barbagallo et al., 2009; Luhrmann et al., 2009; Russell, 2001; Veldurthy et al., 2016; Volpi et al., 2004). She reported that 75 percent of older adults (71 years and older) and 66 percent of older adults with incomes less than 130 percent of the poverty level use dietary supplements, which pose an extra expense but indicate that the nutritional risk of older adults is modifiable with dietary supplement use (Cowan et al., 2018, 2019). Another research gap is that usual nutrient intake from foods is poor among older adults with low incomes, but this group's usual nutrient intake from total sources (food plus dietary supplements) is unknown.

Eicher-Miller explained that some food assistance is available based on income level and sometimes age. One federal program, the Supplemental Nutrition Assistance Program (SNAP), formerly known as the Food Stamp Program, provides monthly benefits to households with income less than or equal to 130 percent of the poverty level. Other programs are community based, such as food pantries that do not have income restrictions and provide foods to local communities. Community meal and meal delivery programs serve older adults aged 60 years and over at reduced or no cost. Recent changes to the Farm Bill will allow SNAP benefits to be used for dietary supplements, which she believes may help meet known nutrient gaps among older adults but could divert this population's limited food-purchasing resources to products that do not provide energy. More information about the characteristics of dietary supplement users and nonusers and their effect on dietary quality in older adults with low incomes is required to inform decision-making for SNAP benefits.

Eicher-Miller described her research study to determine, among U.S. older adults with low incomes, the percentage that have food insecurity and the percentage that use dietary supplements. The study then sought to understand, for each population, its usual nutrient intakes (from food alone and from food plus supplements) and dietary quality. The sample was drawn from NHANES 2007–2016 data on individuals aged 60 years or older with incomes below 130 percent of the poverty line. Among the full sample of 2,347 individuals, nearly 40 percent had low or very low food insecurity, up to about 20 percent were using at least one food assistance program, and close to 60 percent were using dietary supplements.

Eicher-Miller reported that usual nutrient intakes from food were generally poor among the study sample; specifically, at least half of the sample did not meet dietary intake recommendations for six (whole grains, sodium, dairy, fatty acids, and vitamin D) of 10 dietary components examined (Jun et al., 2020). For two nutrients, vitamin D and vitamin E, nearly 100 percent did not meet requirements. Nutrient intake improved when both food and supplement sources were considered. The sample's dietary quality was poor based on the Healthy Eating Index (HEI) score of 58.7 out of 100, and its subscores for individual dietary components within the index were particularly poor for whole grains, sodium, dairy, and fatty acids. When results were stratified to compare dietary supplement users and nonusers, users were more likely to be female, 70 years and older, non-Hispanic White, and of higher educational attainment. Total dietary quality was not significantly different between supplement users and nonusers, she reported, nor was food security status or food assistance use.

Eicher-Miller offered a number of conclusions from the study, beginning with the statement that low income differentiates nutritional risk among older adults. A high prevalence of older adults with low incomes are at risk of inadequate nutrient intakes from foods alone, but dietary supplements play a key role in meeting recommended intakes and are used by about 60 percent of this group. Supplement use greatly affected their nutrition status, and supplements commonly used by the older adult population at large (e.g., calcium) were also the most impactful. Eicher-Miller thought that this supported supplement use to improve situations where low income and food insecurity make it difficult to meet nutrient needs.

Eicher-Miller suggested three research ideas to help close the evidence gap on how to improve nutrient intakes for all older adults, particularly the 40 percent who do not use dietary supplements: examine household resource management and prioritization of foods or supplements, strategies to close the gap between food assistance eligibility and enrollment, and additional characteristics of dietary supplement users and nonusers. Such knowledge could indicate how program and policy changes may support nutrition for older adults with low incomes and food insecurity.

DANISH EXPERIENCES WITH SCREENING

Sussi Friis Buhl, University of Southern Denmark, discussed nutritional challenges among advanced age, self-reliant, community-dwelling adults. She began by noting an important difference between Denmark and other countries: the Danish health care system is publicly financed, primarily through taxes of 37–53 percent. The health care system exists at national, regional, and local levels, and the local level is responsible for many aspects of older adult services, including disease prevention and health promotion, rehabilitation outside of hospitals, home care services, and nursing homes.

One of Denmark's mandated national disease prevention strategies is preventive home visits for older adults, which are offered annually from 82 years or individually planned for those 65 or over who are at risk of low social, psychological, and physical function (Danish Ministry of Social Affairs, 2015). Buhl explained that the aim is to identify older adults at risk of loss of physical function and those who may transfer into settings where more health care services are needed. Healthy foods are promoted and malnutrition risk assessed during the home visits.

Buhl stated that the issue with this advanced age group is that little is known about their nutritional challenges, because adults over 75 are not included in the Danish national dietary survey, and this self-reliant, community-dwelling population is not systematically screened for nutritional status. Protein malnutrition is of interest in this population; European and Nordic dietary recommendations call for higher protein intakes to support optimal health while aging for older compared to younger adults, consistent with global recommendations (Deutz et al., 2014; Nordic Council of Ministers, 2014). If protein intake falls short of requirements or the turnover of protein is not balanced by dietary intake, muscle protein synthesis is reduced and muscle mass can decrease (Tome et al., 2021).

Buhl described a study called "I'm Still Standing" that sought to understand if protein malnutrition is a nutritional challenge in adults of advanced age and if it could be addressed within primary prevention strategies (Buhl et al., 2020). The cross-sectional study included two home visits with self-reliant adults aged 80 years and older. Participants completed a 4-day food record in detail, which was used to calculate protein intake, and underwent assessment of risk factors associated with malnutrition via validated screening tools. Of the 126 participants with completed food records, 54 percent had average protein intake below the European minimum recommended level of 1.0 gram per kilogram of body weight. Participants with low protein intakes were older and more likely to have high BMI and low physical function than those at the recommended intakes. Buhl emphasized that unintentional weight loss did not differ between the two groups, although those with low protein intake more frequently reported reduced appetite and mouth dryness. Using the MNA, 83 percent of participants with low protein intake were categorized as normal nutritional status. Buhl concluded that the results indicate a high prevalence of protein malnutrition in these adults, leading to a study to examine whether population screening during preventive home visits can detect risk factors for low protein intake.

Buhl described the Welfare Innovation in Primary Prevention study's effort to develop and test a screening tool that could identify older adults at risk of losing physical function early (Buhl, 2020, pp. 1-13). It was developed and tested in close collaboration with health care workers and academia. Researchers wanted to know if selected nutrition-related risk factors were associated with accelerated aging or diminished physical function, which they parsed through questions about poor dental status, dysphagia, unintentional weight loss, recent illness, BMI (>27 or <22 kg/m^2), and an assessment tool for physical frailty. Participants were 1,430 older adults with an average age of 81 and nearly 61 percent female. The prevalence of physical frailty was 2.7 percent, although nearly half the sample was pre-frail. One or more nutritional risk factors were self-reported for 60.2 percent, and those that were independently associated with physical pre-frail or frail condition were weight loss, dental status, dysphagia, and high BMI. Moreover, presence of two or more nutritional risk factors was associated with more than a twofold increased risk for pre-frail/frail status.

Buhl highlighted that a major challenge in detecting protein malnutrition via primary prevention programs is that specialized equipment is not available in these settings to estimate muscle mass. Anthropometric measurements are often not feasible within primary prevention, and robust reference ranges do not exist for adults of advanced age, in particular those with coexisting excess weight and reduced muscle mass. Research can inform how to operationalize this in populations with advanced age and high body mass.

PANEL DISCUSSION WITH SPEAKERS

The four speakers answered questions from the workshop's planning committee members and attendees about best practices, knowledge gaps, and research priorities for nutritional screening of older adults. Topics included food insecurity among older adults during the COVID-19 pandemic, screening for malnutrition in federal food assistance programs, stigma associated with participation in those programs, calf circumference as a surrogate for lean body mass, choice of screening tool for different settings, follow-up actions for individuals identified at home visits as having nutritional risks, and gaps and research priorities for screening.

Food Insecurity Among Older Adults
During the COVID-19 Pandemic

Eicher-Miller responded to a question about prevalence of food insecurity during the pandemic. National data are available for 2020 and data on certain segments of time during that year. Overall, data suggest an episodic spike in food insecurity at one point during 2020, but data for the full year suggest that food insecurity rates were relatively unchanged compared with 2019. Eicher-Miller shared that a hypothesis to explain this stability is that quickly implemented changes and flexibilities granted to SNAP and other food assistance programs and the community response of food bank and food pantry support were able to mitigate any spikes. However, data suggest that some racial and ethnic minority groups experienced disproportionately higher rates of food insecurity.

Screening for Malnutrition in Federal Food Assistance Programs

Eicher-Miller explained that SNAP eligibility is based primarily on income and includes certain older U.S. adults with higher incomes than the standard 130 percent poverty threshold cutoff. To her knowledge, the only federal food assistance program that includes a malnutrition screening component, which is offered to participants deemed to be at nutritional risk, is the Special Supplemental Nutrition Program for Women, Infants, and Children. She noted that individuals across the spectrum of BMI can be at risk for malnutrition and added that overweight, obesity, and underweight are prevalent among older adults with low incomes, unlike younger segments of the low-income population, where underweight is less prevalent.

According to Keller, this situation indicates that the metric to detect malnutrition should be not body weight but unintentional weight loss and change in body weight and foods consumed. It is important that screening tools can detect these factors, and she echoed van der Schueren's observation that most screening tools focus on significant weight loss, underweight, and the like, which do not capture the full breadth of upstream factors driving malnutrition.

Stigma Associated with Participation in Federal Food Assistance Programs

Carol Boushey, University of Hawai'i Cancer Center and chair of the workshop planning committee, and Eicher-Miller agreed that they think federal food assistance program participants generally appreciate the opportunity. Eicher-Miller qualified that she has not studied stigma among participants but suggested that some older adults may be reluctant to use these programs out of a desire to be self-reliant. The transition to electronic benefit transfer cards for SNAP benefits was in part due to an attempt to reduce stigma.

Heather Keller, University of Waterloo (UW) and Schlegel-UW Research Institute for Aging, said that Canada does not have an equivalent to SNAP; it has food banks, but older adults do not use these as much as younger adults do, due to location and accessibility. Canada provides a significant advanced age security component that supports food security among older adults, which is the population with the lowest rates of food insecurity.

Keller referenced qualitative research about messaging nutrition risk, reporting that some older adults become offended when told they are at nutrition risk or are malnourished or are in denial. Language sensitivities may be different across countries, and she urged consideration of the language used to convey that nutritional concerns exist and should be addressed.

Calf Circumference as a Surrogate for Lean Body Mass

A planning committee member asked the speakers to describe any evidence to support the use of calf circumference measurements as a surrogate for lean body mass. Jensen replied that validation research has been done and that this measure is easy to use, portable, and practical. He wondered how it compares to other portable measures of muscle in terms of predictive value for lean body mass; it would be a major breakthrough if a portable imaging or ultrasound technique for measuring lean mass were developed and validated for older adults.

A recent GLIM paper promoted calf circumference as a proxy measure for lean body mass, de van der Schueren said, because GLIM is intended to be used worldwide (Barazzoni et al., 2022, pp. 1425–1433). Low-income countries and other countries that want to use GLIM in the community do not have CT or MRI in those settings, so anthropometric measures were added to the phenotypic criteria to enable muscle mass assessment. Keller concurred that calf circumference is easy to measure in the community, requires little training, and is highly correlated with standardized measures of malnutrition, such as the Subjective Global Assessment or MNA.

Calf circumference could be used in preventive home visits in Denmark, Buhl said, given its ease of use in primary prevention. A potential concern is that an increasing number of older adults are both overweight and malnourished, and she wondered if malnutrition is still detectable via calf circumference for them.

Jensen said that malnutrition among older adults with overweight or obesity has become a concern. As an example, he shared that micronutrient deficiencies are common in older Pennsylvanians who have obesity, but screening is not typically conducted for these. On the other hand, he said, screening for unintentional weight loss among older adults with obesity could raise a red flag. Jensen said that he was not aware of any fully validated malnutrition risk screening tools for older adults with overweight or obesity. The GLIM approach is one of few that readily facilitates malnutrition diagnosis among overweight or obese individuals.

Choice of Screening Tool for Different Settings

A workshop attendee asked what screening tool would be best for population studies, home-delivered and congregate meal settings, and assisted-living facilities. The participants in each of those settings are different, Keller pointed out, and therefore so are the malnutrition risk factors, which would call for a different screening tool in each setting. Corish said that according to the MaNuEL project's tool scoring system, those with the highest scores for different settings were the Determine Your Health Checklist (community), NUFFE (rehabilitation), SNAQ (residential care), and MNA and MST (hospital). For a large cohort study, de van der Schueren suggested keeping questions simple and asking about involuntary weight loss and BMI status.

Follow-Up Actions for Individuals with
Nutrition Risks as Identified at Home Visits

Buhl said that Danish health care personnel conduct the preventive health visits for older adults, such as physical or occupational therapists, nurses, or clinical dietitians. The visits are financed by federal tax dollars as part of a preventive strategy; this is a voluntary offer but also a targeted intervention to prevent the need for in-home services or nursing home care.

A new guideline from the Danish health authority is expected soon that will recommend follow-up action if unintentional weight loss is identified during a home visit. She suggested a systematic approach whereby a standardized question about unintentional weight loss is asked at all such visits. Health care staff who conduct the visits cover many topics during the 45 minutes or so, and a specific guideline could help ensure that nutrition is addressed.

An attendee asked Buhl what happens after an individual is identified as having protein insufficiency or other malnutrition. She responded that it depends on where the individual lives, because the municipalities that provide preventive home visits also offer different follow-up strategies to address any conditions identified. Many municipalities have clinical dietitians or other professionals with nutritional expertise, who visit affected individuals to provide dietary advice.

Gaps and Research Priorities for Nutritional Screening

In this era of multiple screening tool options, de van der Schueren said, the next steps are to determine what are the goals of screening, which tools fit those goals, and how screening can best be implemented and connected to interventions to address any abnormalities. Corish concurred and praised GLIM's progress in harmonizing global malnutrition screening efforts, urging further global collaboration to advance progress in the coming decades.

REFERENCES

ASPE (Office of the Assistant Secretary for Planning and Evaluation). 2021. *2021 poverty guidelines for the 48 contiguous states and the District of Columbia.* ASPE.

Bailey, R. L., S. R. Akabas, E. E. Paxson, S. V. Thuppal, S. Saklani, and K. L. Tucker. 2017. Total usual intake of shortfall nutrients varies with poverty among U.S. adults. *Journal of Nutrition Education and Behavior* 49(8):639–646 e633.

Barazzoni, R., G. L. Jensen, M. I. T. Correia, M. C. Gonzalez, T. Higashiguchi, H. P. Shi, S. C. Bischoff, Y. Boirie, F. Carrasco, A. Cruz-Jentoft, and V. Fuchs-Tarlovsky. 2022. Guidance for assessment of the muscle mass phenotypic criterion for the Global Leadership Initiative on Malnutrition (GLIM) diagnosis of malnutrition. *Clinical Nutrition* 41(6):1425–1433.

Barbagallo, M., M. Belvedere, and L. J. Dominguez. 2009. Magnesium homeostasis and aging. *Magnesium Research* 22(4):235–246.

Borkent, J. W., L. T. Schuurman, J. Beelen, J. O. Linschooten, H. H. Keller, A. J. C. Roodenburg, and M. A. E. De van der Schueren. 2020. What do screening tools measure? Lessons learned from SCREEN II and SNAQ(65). *Clinical Nutrition ESPEN* 38:172–177.

Buhl, S. F., A. M. Beck, B. Christensen, and P. Caserotti. 2020. Effects of high-protein diet combined with exercise to counteract frailty in pre-frail and frail community-dwelling older adults: Study protocol for a three-arm randomized controlled trial. *Trials* 21(1):1–13.

Cederholm, T., G. L. Jensen, M. Correia, M. C. Gonzalez, R. Fukushima, T. Higashiguchi, G. Baptista, R. Barazzoni, R. Blaauw, A. Coats, A. Crivelli, D. C. Evans, L. Gramlich, V. Fuchs-Tarlovsky, H. Keller, L. Llido, A. Malone, K. M. Mogensen, J. E. Morley, M. Muscaritoli, I. Nyulasi, M. Pirlich, V. Pisprasert, M. A. E. de van der Schueren, S. Siltharm, P. Singer, K. Tappenden, N. Velasco, D. Waitzberg, P. Yamwong, J. Yu, A. Van Gossum, C. Compher, GLIM Core Leadership Committee, and GLIM Working Group. 2019. GLIM criteria for the diagnosis of malnutrition—A consensus report from the global clinical nutrition community. *Clinical Nutrition* 38(1):19.

Coleman-Jensen, A., M. P. Rabbitt, C. A. Gregory, and A. Singh. 2021. *Household food security in the United States in 2020.* U.S. Department of Agriculture, Economic Research Service.

Cowan, A. E., S. Jun, J. J. Gahche, J. A. Tooze, J. T. Dwyer, H. A. Eicher-Miller, A. Bhadra, P. M. Guenther, N. Potischman, K. W. Dodd, and R. L. Bailey. 2018. Dietary supplement use differs by socioeconomic and health-related characteristics among U.S. adults, NHANES 2011–2014. *Nutrients* 10(8).

Cowan, A. E., S. Jun, J. A. Tooze, H. A. Eicher-Miller, K. W. Dodd, J. J. Gahche, P. M. Guenther, J. T. Dwyer, N. Potischman, A. Bhadra, and R. L. Bailey. 2019. Total usual micronutrient intakes compared to the Dietary Reference Intakes among U.S. adults by food security status. *Nutrients* 12(1).

Danish Ministry of Social Affairs. 2015. Consolidation act on social services. https://english. sm.dk/media/14900/consolidation-act-on-social-services.pdf (accessed September 14, 2022).

Deutz, N. E., J. M. Bauer, R. Barazzoni, G. Biolo, Y. Boirie, A. Bosy-Westphal, T. Cederholm, A. Cruz-Jentoft, Z. Krznaric, K. S. Nair, P. Singer, D. Teta, K. Tipton, and P. C. Calder. 2014. Protein intake and exercise for optimal muscle function with aging: Recommendations from the ESPEN expert group. *Clinical Nutrition* 33(6):929–936.

Guigoz, Y., and B. Vellas. 2021. Nutritional assessment in older adults: MNA® 25 years of a screening tool and a reference standard for care and research; what next? *Journal of Nutrition, Health & Aging* 25(4):528–583.

Hiza, H. A., K. O. Casavale, P. M. Guenther, and C. A. Davis. 2013. Diet quality of Americans differs by age, sex, race/ethnicity, income, and education level. *Journal of the Academy of Nutrition and Dietetics* 113(2):297–306.

Holben, D. H., and A. M. Pheley. 2006. Diabetes risk and obesity in food-insecure households in rural Appalachian Ohio. *Preventing Chronic Disease* 3(3):A82.

Jensen, G. L., K. Kita, J. Fish, D. Heydt, and C. Frey. 1997. Nutrition risk screening characteristics of rural older persons: Relation to functional limitations and health care charges. *American Journal of Clinical Nutrition* 66(4):819–828.

Jensen, G. L., T. Cederholm, M. Correia, M. C. Gonzalez, R. Fukushima, T. Higashiguchi, G. A. de Baptista, R. Barazzoni, R. Blaauw, A. J. S. Coats, A. Crivelli, D. C. Evans, L. Gramlich, V. Fuchs-Tarlovsky, H. Keller, L. Llido, A. Malone, K. M. Mogensen, J. E. Morley, M. Muscaritoli, I. Nyulasi, M. Pirlich, V. Pisprasert, M. de van der Schueren, S. Siltharm, P. Singer, K. A. Tappenden, N. Velasco, D. L. Waitzberg, P. Yamwong, J. Yu, C. Compher, and A. Van Gossum. 2019. GLIM criteria for the diagnosis of malnutrition: A consensus report from the global clinical nutrition community. *Journal of Parenteral and Enteral Nutrition* 43(1):32–40.

Jun, S., A. E. Cowan, A. Bhadra, K. W. Dodd, J. T. Dwyer, H. A. Eicher-Miller, J. J. Gahche, P. M. Guenther, N. Potischman, J. A. Tooze, and R. L. Bailey. 2020. Older adults with obesity have higher risks of some micronutrient inadequacies and lower overall dietary quality compared to peers with a healthy weight, National Health and Nutrition Examination Surveys (NHANES), 2011–2014. *Public Health Nutrition* 23(13):2268–2279.

Kondrup, J., S. P, Allison, M. Elia, B. Vellas, M. Plauth, Educational and Clinical Practice Committee, and European Society of Parenteral and Enteral Nutrition. 2003. ESPEN guidelines for nutrition screening 2002. *Clinical Nutrition* 22(4):415–421.

Leij-Halfwerk, S., M. H. Verwijs, S. van Houdt, J. W. Borkent, P. R. Guaitoli, T. Pelgrim, M. W. Heymans, L. Power, M. Visser, C. A. Corish, M. A. E. de van der Schueren, and MaNuEL Consortium. 2019. Prevalence of protein-energy malnutrition risk in European older adults in community, residential and hospital settings, according to 22 malnutrition screening tools validated for use in adults ≥65 years: A systematic review and meta-analysis. *Maturitas* 126:80–89.

Luhrmann, P. M., R. Bender, B. Edelmann-Schafer, and M. Neuhauser-Berthold. 2009. Longitudinal changes in energy expenditure in an elderly German population: A 12-year follow-up. *European Journal of Clinical Nutrition* 63(8):986–992.

Marshall, E. L. 2010. Examining the relationship between weight, food insecurity, food stamps, and perceived diet quality in school-aged children. *University of Kentucky Master's Theses* (45).

Miller, L. M. S., D. J. Tancredi, L. L. Kaiser, and J. T. Tseng. 2020. Midlife vulnerability and food insecurity: Findings from low-income adults in the U.S. National Health Interview Survey. *PLoS One* 15(7):e0233029.

Nordic Council of Ministers. 2014. *Nordic nutrition recommendations 2012.* https://norden. diva-portal.org/smash/get/diva2:704251/FULLTEXT01.pdf (accessed September 14, 2022).

Pan, L., B. Sherry, R. Njai, and H. M. Blanck. 2012. Food insecurity is associated with obesity among U.S. adults in 12 states. *Journal of the Academy of Nutrition and Dietetics* 112(9):1403–1409.

Posner, B. M., A. M. Jette, K. W. Smith, and D. R. Miller. 1993. Nutrition and health risks in the elderly: The Nutrition Screening Initiative. *American Journal of Public Health* 83(7):972–978.

Power, L., D. Mullally, E. R. Gibney, M. Clarke, M. Visser, D. Volkert, L. Bardon, M. A. E. de van der Schueren, C. A. Corish, and MaNuEL Consortium. 2018. A review of the validity of malnutrition screening tools used in older adults in community and healthcare settings—A MaNuEL study. *Clinical Nutrition ESPEN* 24:1–13.

Power, L., M. A. E. de van der Schueren, S. Leij-Halfwerk, J. Bauer, M. Clarke, M. Visser, D. Volkert, L. Bardon, E. Gibney, C. A. Corish, and MaNuEL Consortium. 2019. Development and application of a scoring system to rate malnutrition screening tools used in older adults in community and healthcare settings—A MaNuEL study. *Clinical Nutrition* 38(4):1807–1819.

Russell, R. M. 2001. Factors in aging that effect the bioavailability of nutrients. *Journal of Nutrition* 131(4 Suppl):1359S-1361S.

Sahyoun, N. R., P. F. Jacques, G. E. Dallal, and R. M. Russell. 1997. Nutrition screening initiative checklist may be a better awareness/educational tool than a screening one. *Journal of the American Dietetic Association* 97(7):760–764.

Seligman, H. K., B. A. Laraia, and M. B. Kushel. 2010. Food insecurity is associated with chronic disease among low-income NHANES participants. *Journal of Nutrition* 140(2):304–310.

Silva, D. F. O., S. Lima, K. C. M. Sena-Evangelista, D. M. Marchioni, R. N. Cobucci, and F. B. Andrade. 2020. Nutritional risk screening tools for older adults with COVID-19: A systematic review. *Nutrients* 12(10).

Tome, D., S. Benoit, and D. Azzout-Marniche. 2021. Protein metabolism and related body function: Mechanistic approaches and health consequences. *Proceedings of the Nutrition Society* 80(2):243–251.

U.S. Census Bureau. 2021. Figure 8. Number in poverty and poverty rate: 1959 to 2020: Current Population Survey, 1960 to 2021 Annual Social and Economic Supplements (CPS ASEC).

Veldurthy, V., R. Wei, L. Oz, P. Dhawan, Y. H. Jeon, and S. Christakos. 2016. Vitamin D, calcium homeostasis and aging. *Bone Research* 4:16041.

Vellas, B., Y. Guigoz, P. J. Garry, F. Nourhashemi, D. Bennahum, S. Lauque, and J. L. Albarede. 1999. The Mini Nutritional Assessment (MNA) and its use in grading the nutritional state of elderly patients. *Nutrition* 15(2):116–122.

Volpi, E., R. Nazemi, and S. Fujita. 2004. Muscle tissue changes with aging. *Current Opinion in Clinical Nutrition and Metabolic Care* 7(4):405–410.

5

Nutritional Policies, Practices, and Challenges That Affect Older Adults

---

BOX 5-1
HIGHLIGHTS[a]

- Few policies exist in terms of educating the medical workforce on nutrition principles and counseling strategies, and most U.S. medical schools do not meet the minimum number of recommended hours for providing nutrition instruction. The Culinary Medicine Specialist Board has developed an eight-module culinary medicine elective that is offered by several U.S. medical schools, and students who take it are four times more likely than those who do not to understand Mediterranean and Dietary Approaches to Stop Hypertension dietary pattern principles and to have a meaningful conversation with patients about these approaches. (Harlan)
- As the pandemic has accelerated the integration of technology into policies and programs offered by aging service providers and community-based programs, opportunities abound to evolve and improve the reach, uptake, and outcomes of aging and nutrition services provided in the community. Despite these technological advances, older adults still desire the high-touch, in-person, in-home services that are at the heart of the Older Americans Act signature programs, such as Meals on Wheels. Responsive, safe, person-centered access to services can be ensured by expanding and scaling effective policy approaches, connecting community-based senior nutrition programs to other service sectors, such as health care, and prioritizing nutrition security. (Akomundo)
- Topics such as food insecurity and social determinants of health are often seen as outside the realms of medicine and health care spending, but advances in payment reform can support and incentivize care transformation

---

that addresses both medical and social needs to advance health equity. Three principles for such reform are to reward reduction of disparities, provide up-front money for investments in infrastructure that addresses social needs, and implement risk-adjusted payment so that safety-net clinics and hospitals are not penalized for caring for more complex patients. (Chin)

- A congressional and regulatory focus on food and nutrition policies that pro-mote availability, accessibility, and affordability of nutritious foods can help address the "triple threat" to older adult health—hunger, food insecurity, and malnutrition—and promote healthy aging. Increasing funding and accessibility of older adult nutrition programs is key, as is increased flexibility for congre-gate meal programs so that they can adapt to the effects of the pandemic. (Blancato)

---

[a]This list is the rapporteurs' summary of points made by the individual speakers identi-fied, and the statements have not been endorsed or verified by the National Academies of Sciences, Engineering, and Medicine. They are not intended to reflect a consensus among workshop participants.

The fourth and final workshop, held May 6, 2022, featured four pre-sentations that highlighted policies, practices, and related challenges that affect older adults, followed by a panel discussion with the speakers. Pre-sentation topics included education policy, food policy, health care payment policy, and the policy landscape.

Elbert Huang, University of Chicago, and Rose Ann DiMaria-Ghalili, Drexel University, co-moderated the session. Huang briefly outlined the role of policy in moving the field toward optimal dietary assessment. The field will determine optimal approaches to nutritional screening and dietary assessment and which are most suitable for community, long-term care, and hospital settings. In his ideal world, screening and assessment would be applied universally and the results translated into targeted nutritional interventions that produce enhanced outcomes for older adults (Figure 5-1).

Huang raised three examples of policy questions that relate to his dia-gram (Figure 5-1). First, who is responsible for delivery of screening and assessment, and how should that workforce be educated? Second, what role should health care and health insurance systems play in both screening and assessment and targeted nutritional interventions? Third, what is the role of federal food assistance programs, and how can they incorporate the latest findings in assessment?

Huang pointed out that multilayered influences beyond individual fac-tors, such as knowledge and preferences, affect food choices, such as vari-ous sociocultural, community, agricultural, government, and even global factors (Mozaffarian et al., 2018). Interest is heightened in nutrition policy;

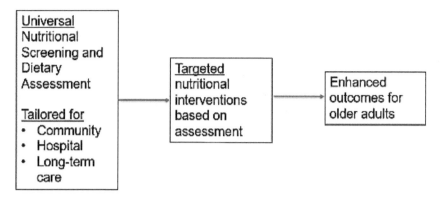

FIGURE 5-1 Ideal world of dietary assessment.
SOURCE: Presented by Elbert Huang on May 6, 2022.

he shared the example that the Biden-Harris administration announced the White House Conference on Hunger, Nutrition, and Health for September 2022.[1] This is only the second-ever White House conference on these topics since 1969, and it will release a national strategy for ending hunger and improving nutrition and physical activity by 2030 so that fewer Americans experience diet-related chronic diseases.

EDUCATION POLICY: TEACHING ABOUT FOOD AND NUTRITION IN MEDICINE

Timothy Harlan, George Washington University, discussed nutrition education for health care professionals beyond registered dietitians (e.g., physicians, residents, medical and nursing students). Many physicians think that their patients do not listen to them, he said, when it comes to healthy lifestyle counseling. But evidence suggests that patients listen to physician advice about health behavior change (Kreuter et al., 2000), and when physicians disclose healthy personal behaviors, it improves their credibility and ability to motivate patients to adopt healthy habits (Frank et al., 2000). In other words, patients are more likely to follow physicians who "talk the talk" and "walk the walk." This principle is borne out in the smoking cessation literature, which indicates that prevalence of physician smoking fell from nearly 60 percent in 1945 to around 5 percent in 1985 as the health

---

[1]   https://health.gov/our-work/nutrition-physical-activity/white-house-conference-hunger-nutrition-and-health#:~:text=The%202022%20White%20House%20Conference,close%20the%20disparities%20surrounding%20them (accessed September 14, 2022).

effects became apparent (Smith, 2008). The decrease in smoking prevalence among the public is not as drastic but follows a similar trajectory, and Medicare reimburses physicians to discuss smoking cessation.

Harlan said that despite the evidence that suggests the positive effect of health care professional counseling on patient behavior change few policies exist in terms of educating the workforce in nutrition principles and counseling strategies. He referenced a report on nutrition education in medical schools (National Research Council Committee on Nutrition in Medical Education, 1985), which was one of the first attempts to issue policy recommendations. It recommended a minimum of 25–30 classroom hours in nutrition during the preclinical years; in 2002, the National Institutes of Health (NIH) set forth a nutrition curriculum guide that describes what physicians and health care professionals need to know to be equipped to discuss diet and dietary behaviors with patients (Curriculum Committee of the Nutrition Academic Award Program, 2002). Nonetheless, a 2010 survey of accredited U.S. medical schools indicated that most do not meet that minimum recommendation (Adams et al., 2006). A standardized nutrition curriculum for medical schools does not exist, although the Liaison Committee on Medical Education (the accrediting body for educational programs at U.S. and Canadian schools of medicine) and Association of American Medical Colleges (Kushner et al., 2014) have also issued recommendations. Each medical school sets its own curriculum; he shared an example from his own institution, where approximately 1 percent of the objectives required of first- and second-year students are related to nutrition. Harlan pointed out that nutrition encompasses a broad range of topics, such as physiologic aspects (e.g., digestion, absorption, and metabolism) and dietary assessment and behavior change counseling.

Harlan mentioned a nonprofit organization, the Culinary Medicine Specialist Board, a group of several dozen medical schools and partner sites with a vision to "empower healthier lifestyles and reshape the course of chronic disease in America by integrating the science of medicine into culinary tradition" (Stauber et al., 2022, pp. 214-220). The core of this initiative is community programming delivered directly to patients, which includes hands-on cooking classes at teaching kitchens in medical schools and hospitals.

Another component is medical student programming on nutrition and culinary topics; it empowers students to be what he called "force multipliers" by providing the opportunity to help deliver the community programming. First- and second-year students in 10 medical schools are required to take a 3-hour course that introduces them to nutrition, cooking techniques, and techniques for patient communication about dietary behaviors (Pang et al., 2019). Hands-on cooking classes combine case- and team-based learning that connect the physiological aspects of nutrition to the food-related patient conversations. An eight-module culinary medicine elective is also available for students interested in additional coursework; it includes 33 modules that schools may include. These cover a range of foundational topics and nutrition for various life stages and conditions (e.g., heart disease, diabetes, celiac disease, food allergies, HIV, and eating disorders), which emphasizes that nutrition spans a wide variety of topics. He highlighted a module on geriatrics, admitting that it is relatively short and could be expanded substantially.

Harlan discussed the Mediterranean-style diet, which is a focus of the programming for both community members and medical professionals. It is emphasized based on evidence supporting its effectiveness for weight loss (Sacks et al., 2009), reduced risk of cardiovascular disease events (de Lorgeril et al., 1999), and positive outcomes for a number of other common chronic diseases. Based on evidence indicating that patients in the highest tertile of diet scores experienced significantly lower risk of all-cause mortality compared to patients with lower scores (Trichopoulou et al., 2003), program participants are encouraged to improve their scores by consuming more vegetables, legumes, fruits and nuts, whole grains, and seafood; better-quality oils and fats; and less dairy and meat. Medical students learn how to administer a 24-hour dietary recall, assess the results, and provide counseling to help improve a patient's scores.

Harlan said that programming is also being implemented at culinary schools, based on the impact potential of educating culinarians in how to deliver high-quality, nutrient-rich foods that positively affect health. In addition, programming is available for practicing health care professionals, such as continuing medical education courses, a 60-credit-hour Certified Culinary Medicine Specialist program, and an annual Culinary Medicine Conference. Standardized policies on integrating these topics in medical education do not exist, but he recommended this.

Harlan shared 7 years of data collected to assess the effectiveness of the culinary medicine elective (Leong et al., 2014). It includes 25 core competencies, and students were assessed for their level of improvement in demonstrating each one compared to a control group of nonparticipants. The first year of data indicated a statistically insignificant improvement in most competencies. After rebuilding the courseware, the results dramatically improved for the second and third years. A key factor was involving the students, to understand what they needed to succeed. The program had additional learnings as more medical schools implemented it and contributed results data, and by the seventh year, participants satisfactorily achieved all 25 competencies. Participants are four times more likely to understand Mediterranean or DASH diet principles and have a meaningful conversation with patients about these approaches.

Harlan said that the programming for community members has been found to improve Mediterranean diet scores, attitudes toward cooking, and healthy eating habits, and likelihood of engaging in positive dietary behaviors, with 3 years of data on approximately 500 participants indicating that scores improved notably after the revision (Stauber et al., 2022). In a randomized trial of families, a six-module series was delivered to improve parents' and children's scores. Dramatic improvements were observed compared to a control group, and grocery store receipts were used to project that a family of four would save almost $6,000 per year.

Harlan briefly raised the issue of reimbursement for health care services, which is key when it comes to health care professionals providing nutritional counseling for a range of conditions. He estimated that more than half of patients present for a diet-related condition or disease, and even those who do not will have questions about food. Despite the high importance of food to many patients, medical professionals, outside of dietitians, are not explicitly reimbursed for counseling or guidance.

FOOD POLICY: MEALS ON WHEELS

Ucheoma Akobundu, Meals on Wheels, began with an overview of the national association; it has a network of 5,000+ local and community-based organizations (CBOs) dedicated to addressing social isolation and hunger among older adults. It serves virtually every U.S. community and has more than two million staff and volunteers who deliver nutritious meals and conduct friendly visits and safety checks to enable recipients to live nourished lives with independence and dignity. The national association provides expertise, funding, leadership, education, research, and advocacy support to empower and strengthen local organizations and their staff of aging services, nutrition and food service management, and social service professionals.

Akobundu said that older adults proactively reach out to local Meals on Wheels programs and are screened for nutrition risk and assessed for nutrition needs before receiving services. This helps ensure that services align with their personal lifestyle and culture and any medical needs. Screening is conducted by generalist staff and volunteers, but more specialized nutrition education, counseling, and dietary supplements are provided by registered dietitians.

Akobundu discussed opportunities for policy actions to support nutrition in light of the pandemic's effects on both national and community issues, such as availability of and access to safe and nutritious food, health and nutrition services and interventions, and social support. These challenges have exposed opportunities for reinvention and reimagination in both policy and programmatic areas, which has resulted in targeted, smart policy changes that allow food assistance and nutrition services to flow to older adults most in need. Such changes impacted food production, processing, marketing, and distribution, to promote greater equity among vulnerable groups and provide improved food accessibility and availability.

Akobundu discussed the food policy landscape that governs these services, focusing on the Older Americans Act (OAA).[2] It is a partially federally funded, state-administered social services program to assist older adults and their families, it undergirds Meals on Wheels services nationwide. The act includes establishing an "Aging Network," composed of federal, state, and local agencies to plan and provide services that help individuals to live independently in their homes and communities. This network develops programming for populations with the greatest social and economic need, particularly those who have low incomes, are of minority racial/ethnic backgrounds, reside in rural areas, have limited English proficiency, or are at risk for malnutrition and institutionalization.

Akobundu explained that within OAA, Title III-C (the nutrition services program)[3] aims to reduce hunger, food insecurity, and malnutrition; promote socialization; and improve the health and well-being of older adults by helping them access nutrition and other disease prevention and health promotion services, delaying the onset of adverse outcomes. Since OAA's establishment in 1972, it had three reauthorizations that changed its focus and funding priorities in response to evolving social, demographic, and economic conditions. The first phase focused on life-enhancing or age-mitigating services, pursued mainly through congregate dining programs and home-delivered meal services. In the 1980s, the focus shifted to mitigating vulnerability; in the 1990s, it became integrating care and chronic disease management. Akobundu predicted a focus on integrating technology, noting that "seismic challenges" from the pandemic have accelerated the Aging Network's pivot to technology adoption.

Akobundu elaborated on these challenges, such as shelter-in-place requirements, closing of congregate dining sites, loss of access to senior centers where older adults received services, the impact of social distancing, and reduced home visits. The resulting focus on technology provides opportunities to better support, evolve, and accelerate how aging and nutrition services are provided in the community, leading to positive effects on reach, uptake, and outcomes. For example, technological approaches can facilitate collection of nutrition assessment information in homes and communities by Meals on Wheels program staff and nutrition professionals. Despite these advances, Akobundu emphasized the value of the high-touch,

---

[2] https://uscode.house.gov/view.xhtml?path=/prelim@title42/chapter35&edition=prelim (accessed September 14, 2022).

[3] https://acl.gov/sites/default/files/programs/2019-01/AoA_Issue_Brief_Food_Sources.pdf (accessed September 14, 2022).

in-person, in-home services that are at the heart of OAA and still desired by older adults.

Poverty, social isolation, food insecurity, and disability were challenges for older adults prior to the pandemic and worsened in its wake. Food insecurity among older adults rose from 2.8 to 4.9 percent between 2019 and 2020 (Kinderknecht et al., 2022), and Meals on Wheels programs reported delivering an average of up to 100 percent more meals weekly during 2020. Many older adults, particularly those with physical limitations, had to quickly learn new ways of preparing food, navigating the loss of employment and/or transportation, and adhering to stay-at-home orders while also avoiding exposure to the virus. Akobundu highlighted present challenges, including rising food and gas prices, supply chain issues, hiring and retaining sufficient staff, and a lack of registered community dietitians with expertise in geriatric nutrition.

Akobundu described how Meals on Wheels pivoted early in the pandemic to adapt services to safely meet client needs. Almost all programs changed how services were provided, such as reworking home-delivered meal options and logistics. About half of them tapped local partnerships to help fill gaps and provide emergency meals, and a similar proportion served congregate meal clients in alternative formats, such as grab-and-go, drive-thru, or curbside pick-up. She added that more than half developed opportunities to address social isolation.

With respect to policy pivots during COVID-19, Akobundu listed responses such as expanding eligibility and enrollment criteria to serve more people, decreasing administrative burdens, and facilitating greater access to nutrition services. As an example, she recalled that the Administration for Community Living leveraged flexibilities that were already in statute to ensure that programs could expand to reach older adults in need, such as shifting models to grab-and-go services that could continue to use existing funding streams. Another example is a Coronavirus Aid, Relief, and Economic Security Act provision[4] that enables transferring funding from one service stream to another while bypassing usual administrative processes.

Akobundu shared evidence on the pandemic's impact on older adult dietary intakes, nutrition status, and food security, noting that COVID-19 mitigation policies and practices results in a shift in how food is accessed and consumed. Recent systematic reviews suggest that older adults' food access, diet quality, and nutritional status were maintained or even improved during the pandemic, but these results are not consistent within or across studies (Nicklett et al., 2021). Furthermore, local providers across the Meals

---

[4] https://www.kff.org/coronavirus-covid-19/issue-brief/the-coronavirus-aid-relief-and-economic-security-act-summary-of-key-health-provisions (accessed September 14, 2022).

on Wheels network report food access constraints and negative impacts on their nutritional status.

Akobundu suggested that a shared advocacy agenda includes doubling federal funding for OAA nutrition programs, which are a "proven antidote" to loneliness, hunger, and malnutrition. She also appealed for advancing policies and innovations that support community-based nutrition programs as they strive to serve more older adults and strengthening and expanding the broader network of nutrition and social programs—especially within the charitable sector—that provide vital services and assistance to older adults and their families. She urged policies that support an infusion of focused, targeted funding, programming, time, and outreach effectively used by CBOs to meet the nutrition and well-being needs of older adults.

Akobundu underscored that pandemic-driven food insecurity and hunger are likely to persist as society moves into a post-pandemic era. Older adults will continue to need responsive, safe, person-centered access to services that support their nutrition and wellness needs, and she listed three strategies for addressing these needs during the "next normal." First is to continue expanding effective policy approaches and scaling them in different areas of the country. Second is to "build bridges to build a bigger table," by expanding connections to community-based senior nutrition programs to other service sectors. Health care providers are often in a position to regularly monitor food insecurity in patients, for example, and make referrals to community-based services to meet identified patient needs. Third is to prioritize nutrition security to mitigate the risk of malnutrition among older adults.

HEALTH CARE PAYMENT POLICY: NEW OPPORTUNITIES TO USE MEDICARE DOLLARS TO ADDRESS NUTRITION AND SOCIAL DETERMINANTS OF HEALTH

Marshall Chin, University of Chicago, discussed new opportunities to use health care payment policy levers to address nutrition and social determinants of health. He began by referencing data on the U.S. total health service expenditures, which make up more than half of the country's gross domestic product (GDP). This makes the United States an outlier compared to many other Organisation for Economic Co-operation and Development (OECD) countries, he pointed out, where social service expenditures are a majority of the GDP (Bradley et al., 2011). Chin noted a tension and bias in medicine and health care because topics such as food insecurity and social determinants of health are seen as outside the realm of medicine and health care spending.

Most consumer advocacy groups have traditionally focused on improving access to health care (i.e., access to and expansion of health insurance coverage), although more recently, they have expanded their efforts to include quality of care and payment policy, recognizing that both levers are powerful in terms of the flow of health care dollars. Although these two topics are a little arcane, he pointed out that "this is where a lot of the action is emerging" with respect to the potential to impact food insecurity and social determinants of health among older adults. He urged attendees to understand how these and other payment policy levers could affect food and added that the levers also interact with each other and should not be viewed in isolation.

Chin provided context for his presentation's frame of health equity and social determinants of health. He shared the World Health Organization (WHO) definition of equity, noting its nod to social justice: "Equity is the absence of avoidable or remediable differences among groups of people, whether those groups are defined socially, economically, demographically, or geographically. Health inequities therefore involve more than inequality with respect to health determinants, access to the resources needed to improve and maintain health or health outcomes. They also entail a failure to avoid or overcome inequalities that infringe on fairness and human rights norms."[5] He shared an illustration (Figure 5-2) that depicts the difference between providing the same solution to diverse individuals versus providing individually tailored solutions to meet their different needs and maximize their potential.

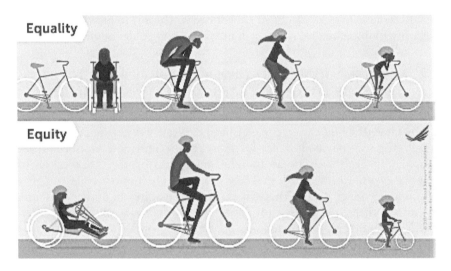

FIGURE 5-2 Illustrated comparison of equality and equity.
SOURCE: Presented by Marshall Chin on May 6, 2022 (Robert Wood Johnson Foundation, 2017).

---

[5] https://www.who.int/health-topics/health-equity#tab=tab_1 (accessed September 14, 2022).

Chin described a framework for advancing health equity (Figure 5-3). He referenced the right side of the framework, which emphasizes payment reform that supports and incentivizes care transformation to advance health equity. He also noted the importance of cross-sectional partnerships to address medical and social drivers of health. He underscored that if advancing health equity is to become a reality, actors must be intentional and commit to the mission of maximizing health among diverse individuals and populations. The classic route in health care is to examine one's data to assess whether a disparate outcome has occurred, conduct a root cause analysis to identify why the disparity exists, and design and implement specific care interventions that address the root causes. Creating a culture of equity is of paramount importance, which includes understanding one's own personal biases and identifying system structures that bias against and oppress marginalized populations. All of these things affect individual and population health as well as health care equity.

WHO defines social determinants of health as "the conditions in which people are born, grow, live, work, and age. These circumstances are shaped by the distribution of money, power, and resources at global, national, and local levels. The social determinants of health are mostly responsible for health inequities, the unfair and avoidable differences in health status seen within and between countries."[6] Chin observed a growing recognition that social drivers of health are very powerful causes of inequities in health outcomes.

Chin referenced his work with the Robert Wood Johnson Foundation's Advancing Health Equity program, which works with state Medicaid agencies, Medicaid managed care organizations, and health care organizations to achieve health equity. The program has a Health Care Payment Learning & Action Network, an active group of several hundred public and private health care leaders dedicated to providing thought leadership, strategic direction, and ongoing support to accelerate the U.S. health care system's adoption of alternative payment models for Medicare and Medicaid. A theme of that work is that the field needs to do a better job of connecting the dots in terms of advancing payment reform that supports and incentivizes care transformation to address medical and social needs and advance health equity.

Chin said that the predominant U.S. health care system is a fee-for-service approach; payment is rendered for individual services, which incentivizes service volume. A shift toward value-based payment is occurring, which rewards the quality—instead of the quantity—of health care services

---

[6] https://www.who.int/westernpacific/activities/taking-action-on-the-social-determinants-of-health#:~:text=Social%20determinants%20of%20health%20are,themselves%20influenced%20by%20policy%20choices (accessed September 14, 2022).

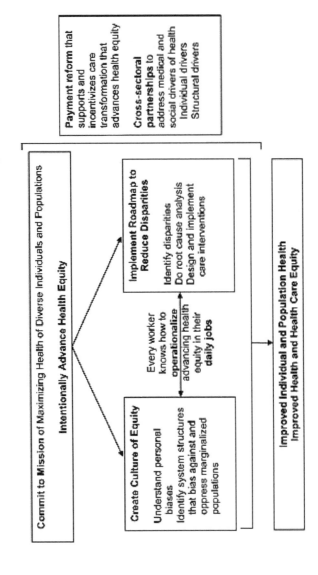

FIGURE 5-3 Framework for advancing health equity.
SOURCE: Presented by Marshall Chin on May 6, 2022 (Chin, 2020).

and health outcomes. The word "value" is embedded in both health outcomes and cost, and alternative payment models promote both value and cost efficiency. Organizations take on financial risk to deliver high-quality care at lower costs; he cited accountable care organizations (ACOs) as an example. ACOs are responsible for the health and costs of a predetermined population of patients, and the rewards and penalties for meeting quality and cost metrics are built into the system. This model is very different from the fee-for-service model, which can be described simply as "the more you do, the more money you get."

Chin listed three principles for the aforementioned payment reform: reward reduction of disparities, provide up-front money for investments in infrastructure (e.g., to address social determinants of health), and implement risk-adjusted payment for the safety net. The rationale for the third principle is that because safety-net clinics and hospitals care for patients with a higher medical and social risk, they would otherwise be penalized for taking care of patients with more challenging health issues, which may cost more.

Chin elaborated on the differences between prospective and retrospective payment models, noting that the latter reward and incentivize reducing disparities and advancing health equity. An example is pay-for-performance, which rewards the outcome rather than providing payment up front (prospective payment). For example, up-front payment may be capitated payments, global budgets, shared savings, or per-member per-month, and he underscored that the basic framework is that the money is available for various uses, which could include addressing social determinants of health, providing the infrastructure and workforce (e.g., community health workers, information technology systems to track equity metrics) for interventions.

Chin raised a series of questions to ask about payment. First, what is being incentivized (or at financial risk)? The most powerful systems are the ones where the total costs of care are at risk. If a health system is responsible for the total cost of care for a given geographic population, it is incentivized to invest in addressing the social determinants of health to keep people healthy and out of the hospital. A related question is the magnitude of the incentive or financial risk. A third question is what patients and populations the health system is responsible for. A fourth is about the appropriate payment targets to advance health equity such as reaching a particular benchmark of achievement, attaining a certain level of improvement in a given metric, or reducing disparities based on a predetermined measure of success. It gets more complicated when one begins to examine alternative payment models, which entail more complicated frameworks. However, these frameworks boil down to the three principles of payment system, payment structures, and process for measuring and rewarding performance.

Chin shared a series of examples of alternative payment models. The first is the Center for Medicare & Medicaid Services (CMS) ACO realizing equity, access, and community health model, which developed a health equity plan that identified disparities in patient outcomes and identified specific actions to mitigate those disparities. This model is a redesign of the CMS Global and Professional Direct Contracting Model in response to new government priorities, which include a commitment to advancing health equity, stakeholder feedback, and participant experience. The purpose is to improve health care for people with Medicare through "better care coordination, reaching and connecting health care providers and beneficiaries, including those beneficiaries who are underserved."[7] They needed to adjust certain health equity benchmarks to better support care delivery and coordination for those in underserved communities, which has required collecting beneficiary-reported demographic and social needs data.

Chin cited another example of alternative payment models, state Medicaid plans, explaining that each state has contracting arrangements with Medicaid managed care organizations. Oregon is the most advanced state, as it is on version 2.0 of what it calls a "coordinated care organization" (McConnell, 2016). This is essentially a network of ACOs with risk-adjusted global budgets and bonuses for meeting performance metrics. Health-related services include flexible services, such as community benefit initiatives, that address social determinants of health, which could include food insecurity. Screening for social determinants is an incentive metric, with requirements to invest in social determinants of health and equity and increase community investment. With this financial flexibility and incentive structure, Oregon has found that more money is spent on health-related services for community benefit (e.g., housing, food security, community capacity building) than the traditional services for individual benefit. Challenges include burdensome reporting and lack of adequate data systems for tracking, measuring, and linking health and social needs, referrals, and feedback.

Chin cited Minnesota's Medicaid plans, which require formal, sustainable partnerships between health care organizations and CBOs, such as food banks. The state's plans have focused on screening, referral, eligibility, assessment, service delivery, and coordination in linking social needs and health care (Martinson et al., 2006). In Massachusetts, contracts are required between ACOs and CBOs. The state assesses health-related social needs of the enrolled population, the available community resources, and gaps in community services (Kaye, 2021). Payment is adjusted for social risk, with incentives to address social determinants via partnerships with CBOs and flexible services. He raised two challenges of linking clinical and

---

[7] https://innovation.cms.gov/innovation-models/aco-reach (accessed September 14, 2022).

community sectors: a fear of health care stakeholders using their muscle in non-health-care spaces (where he suggested they are better suited as partners) and the difficulty of aligning incentives and implementing common metrics across sectors such as housing, criminal justice, and health care.

Local initiatives to improve population health and advance equity through partnerships with community organizations must be viewed within the context of the wider policy challenges, Chin advised, which involve overall health care financing policies and global payment models.

He ended with a quote about caring for diverse populations in current society: "Clinicians must have self-insight and true understanding of heterogeneous patients, knowledge of evidence-based interventions, ability to adapt messaging and approaches, and facility with systems change and advocacy. Advancing health equity requires both science and art; evidence-based roadmaps and stories that guide the journey to better outcomes; judgment that informs how to change the behavior of patients, providers, communities, organizations, and policy makers; and passion and a moral mission to serve humanity" (Chin, 2021).

THE BIG PICTURE AND NEW LEGISLATION

Bob Blancato, Defeat Malnutrition Today coalition, maintained that, in light of the clear connections between dietary intake and health, a focus on older adult nutrition is needed to help achieve healthier aging. He urged a congressional and regulatory focus on what he called the "triple threat" to older adult health: hunger, food insecurity, and malnutrition. The Defeat Malnutrition Today coalition comprises more than 100 organizations and stakeholders that recognize that malnutrition is a key indicator and vital sign of older adult health.

Recent legislation for older adult nutrition has been dominated by responses to the COVID-19 pandemic, such as four emergency funding bills passed by Congress between March 2020 and March 2021; $1.6 billion was provided for OAA as the program underwent its biggest conversion in its 50-year history. One indicator of this conversion is that before the pandemic, 66 percent of older adults served received meals in congregate settings. By the first month of the pandemic, more than 90 percent of them were receiving home-bound or grab-and-go meals, leading to major increases in demand and cost (Blancato and Whitmire, 2021). The emergency funding bills helped address this situation, particularly given rising costs of food and gas, both of which are central to older adult food programs. The bills also supported other nutrition programs that serve older adults, such as SNAP and the Commodity Supplemental Food Program.

Blancato discussed new legislation that will provide funding for fiscal year (FY) 2023 (which begins October 1, 2022, for the federal government).

He noted that the funds included in the emergency spending bills passed for FY 2022 were intended to last through the end of the COVID-19 public health emergency but may run out sooner, and any significant funding reduction levels will lead to a "service cliff" in nutrition programs for older adults nationwide, whereby recipients would lose access to meals. Therefore, a legislative focus is funding for FY 2023 and advocacy groups (e.g., Meals on Wheels America, National Association of Nutrition and Aging Services Programs) are seeking doubled funding for OAA nutrition programs. Funding and increasing accessibility of nutrition programs is key, especially when it comes to directing older adults to programs to which they are entitled. Despite progress in this area, eligible older adults have low SNAP participation; only 42 percent of them participate, compared to 82 percent of eligible persons in the general population (Gray and Cunnyngham, 2016).

Blancato highlighted that advocacy groups are also seeking increased flexibility in meal programs. The pandemic funding increased reimbursement and flexibility for the OAA Congregate Meal Program, but it follows firm guidelines, including low reimbursement rates, strictly balanced meals (i.e., little flexibility to accommodate different dietary preferences, such as vegetarian or kosher), providing only one-third of daily meal requirements (although this stipulation was waived with the emergency pandemic funding), prohibiting food to leave the room, and restricting innovation of the congregate meal space. Increasing flexibility in these areas can increase accessibility of congregate programs as they reopen. Examples of such flexibilities include evaluating and increasing reimbursement rates more frequently, increasing options for meals to fit special dietary needs and/ or accommodate specific preferences (e.g., cultural preferences), adding options for additional servings or take-home meals, modernizing meal spaces and meal options, and making grab-and-go options permanent.

Blancato mentioned the relationships between nutrition and other issues that affect older adults: falls, mental health, and elder abuse. Malnutrition and low body weight are significant risk factors for falls, and rates of depression among older adults increase with age. One-quarter of adults 65 years and older are considered to be socially isolated, which increases the risk of premature death more than smoking, obesity, and inactivity. Social isolation also increases risk of elder abuse, especially self-neglect and financial abuse (NASEM, 2020). The OAA nutrition programs are more than just a meal—they are a source of social and community connection; provide screenings that can help identify malnutrition, food insecurity, fall risk, isolation, and mental health issues; and promote evidence-based disease prevention and health promotion programs to help improve health and well-being and reduce disease and injury.

Blancato discussed regulatory developments that relate to older adult nutrition. A major opportunity to improve care for malnourished older adults in hospitals is the Global Malnutrition Composite Score,[8] a quality measure that was included in the proposed rule for the CMS Inpatient Prospective Payment System and endorsed by the National Quality Forum. The measure calculates the average of the performance scores of four components of the electronic quality measure for people 65 and older: malnutrition screening, nutrition assessment for risk of malnutrition, appropriate malnutrition diagnosis, and nutrition care plan documentation in the medical record for malnourished individuals. To illustrate how this measure would benefit both older adults and hospitals, Blancato reported that malnutrition is estimated to affect more than 30 percent of hospitalized adults but diagnosed in only 9 percent (Barker et al., 2011). Malnourished patients experience poor health outcomes and burden the health care system with higher hospitalization costs, higher readmission rates, and longer average length of stay (Barker et al., 2011), which is why advocates for older adult nutrition want the Global Malnutrition Composite Score quality measure to be included in the final rule.

Blancato circled back to the White House Conference on Hunger, Nutrition, and Health. According to the legislation that paved the way for the conference (H.R.5724), its purpose is to develop a road map to end hunger and improve nutrition by 2030 and to review existing and cross-departmental strategies and consider new approaches to improve health by eliminating hunger, reducing prevalence of chronic diseases, and improving access to and consumption of nutritious foods in accordance with the Dietary Guidelines for Americans. Blancato added that the 2025–2030 edition of the guidelines is anticipated to include a focus on nutritional guidance for older adults (GAO, 2019), and he hoped that the conference will give adequate attention to older adults' unique nutrition needs and dietary assessment considerations. He recalled that based on his experience as a participant in four White House conferences on aging, they can produce recommendations that become the basis for new legislation.

Blancato also touched on Senate bill 1536, the Medical Nutrition Therapy Act of 2021. It would expand the conditions eligible for medical nutrition therapy coverage under Medicare (which covers diabetes and renal disease only) and therefore expand access for more patients to see a registered dietitian to receive medical nutrition therapy counseling. The bill was included in a major House of Representatives bill (H.R.7585) introduced at the end of April 2022 (Health Equity and Accountability Act of 2022).

Blancato asserted that access to nutrition is a public health issue and called for national and state public health goals to address malnutrition,

---

[8] https://www.eatrightpro.org/practice/quality-management/quality-initiatives/global-malnutrition-composite-score (accessed September 14, 2022).

particularly for older adults. Such goals should be part of Healthy People 2030 and be included in year-to-year state plans under OAA. An expanded evidence base on older adult nutrition needs is also needed, along with increased NIH funding for such research, especially evidence on malnutrition's effect on health equity and health outcomes.

Blancato shifted to nutrition security and promotion of nutrition through the life span. In a 2021 *JAMA* Viewpoint article, nutrition security was defined as having "consistent access, availability, and affordability of foods and beverages that promote well-being and prevent (and if needed, treat) disease" (Mozaffarian et al., 2021). The article suggested that prioritizing nutrition security could address a gap in clinical and public health screening tools for food insecurity: a lack of assessment of diet quality or nutrition. It added that "[i]n recognition of the rapid increase in the prevalence of several diet-related diseases and longstanding racial disparities in access to nutritional foods and diet conditions, it is time to embrace the concept of nutrition security." Blancato endorsed this statement, adding that food deserts are an example of the kind of disparity in food access that should be eliminated. In terms of nutrition throughout the life course, access to and affordability of nutrition solutions is important for all generations. One solution is to change pricing policies so that nutrient-dense foods are less expensive relative to nutrient-poor foods, and another is to promote nutrition education during childhood and adolescence, given that many chronic conditions in older adults can be prevented with proper nutrition earlier in life.

Blancato emphasized that sound nutrition is vital for physical and mental health, and he urged a focus on policies that neither reward nor subsidize poor nutrition but instead promote the availability, accessibility, and affordability of nutrient-dense foods.

PANEL DISCUSSION WITH SPEAKERS

The four speakers answered questions from the workshop's planning committee members and attendees about topics that included connecting the dots between health care and community services; meeting the nutrition needs of frail, older adults; legislation and funding mechanisms to address the needs of the oldest old; and key takeaways for health care providers.

Connecting the Dots Between Health
Care and Community Services

Chin responded to a question about how to close the loops of screening for health and social needs in health care and community settings. A goal for health care is to be able to refer patients to CBOs that can address social needs identified in the health care setting. To be successful, health care needs to have a database of relevant community partners and a feedback loop by which the provider could be informed of whether the patient acted on the referral to the CBO. This has been a challenge in practice, although regional demonstration projects have been undertaken and are being evaluated. Despite a lot to learn about how to do this well, Chin said that it is a step in the right direction of coordinated care systems and care transformations that lead to better outcomes.

Blancato shared his observation that private equity firms have inserted themselves into the traditional information and referral space, which is a problem when they bypass existing community-based structures (e.g., 2-1-1s) that have been doing referrals for a long time and already have databases and experience. He suggested building better alliances and communication channels between health care and community-based entities. Akobundu agreed and added that it has been a challenge to break out of the siloes that have prevented effective bidirectional communication to document patient needs. She called for incentives for building an infrastructure that enables these clinical and community linkages.

In response to a follow-up question about connecting the dots at the federal level, Blancato indicated that the connections between federally funded health care and community programs are inadequate. Medicare Advantage is moving deeper into nonmedical supplemental services at the community level, including nutrition, which may create an opportunity for closer linkages to programs like Meals on Wheels.

Chin suggested that systems are set up to be relatively siloed, such that health care or any other sector is designed to respond to incentive structures and metrics for rewards and accountability within its own space rather than thinking about what is best for each patient. A challenge of promoting cross-sector collaboration is the need to establish commonly aligned metrics and incentives, which he characterized as a relatively uncharted space but also a "huge frontier" for advancing health equity.

Meeting the Nutrition Needs of Frail Adults of Advanced Age

The Meals on Wheels network takes pride in providing meals that are responsive to its population's needs, Akobundu said; older adults receive an initial nutrition screening and have access to more in-depth opportunities for evaluation of their lifestyle, religious, medical, and cultural needs. Those needs are met to the extent possible in partnership with the program, so that each individual receives the optimal set of nutrition services. Sometimes programs can also provide assistive devices to support the needs of frail older adults, so they can better manage mealtimes at home.

Legislation and Funding Mechanisms to
Address the Needs of the Oldest Old

In response to a question about future legislative opportunities, Blancato said that the Administration for Community Living administers OAA and can instruct what programming is added to state or area plans. If nutrition is lacking in a particular geographic area, that it is the advocate's job to lobby for greater emphasis on nutrition in future plans.

Chin observed a difference in how funding streams work in emergency versus nonemergency situations. Emergency funds typically use existing mechanisms to funnel money, because it is hard to create a new funding mechanism during an emergency. He suggested that the reason some of the initial CARES Act funding for health care organizations was not necessarily weighted toward the greatest needs or most vulnerable populations was that it had to go through existing channels. Chin suggested that more integrative funding streams could be established to better support the linkages between medical and social needs and facilitate the bidirectional flow of information between these sectors.

Key Takeaways for Health Care Providers

In DiMaria-Ghalili's view, the take-home message is the importance of training all health care providers across the care continuum to screen older adults for nutrition risk, including during office and home care visits. Screening should also occur at both hospital admission and discharge, and the latter is important for indicating what services a patient might need at home.

Akobundu built on DiMaria-Ghalili's contribution, commenting that much of health care happens outside of the walls of health care institutions. She urged building a bigger loop of clinical and community partners who can play different roles in intervening, screening, assessing, and transferring information. As an example, she suggested that dentists could ask older adults about their nutrition habits and refer to food and nutrition assistance programs.

According to Harlan, the first step is to make food part of conversations between health care providers and patients. Physicians are trained to conduct physical exams and collect a family medical history, and he posited that a dietary history might be more important than a family medical history. Food conversations can broach the topic of food security by asking where a patient gets food. He shared a web link for a free CME course on food security.

Chin suggested that advocacy is inherent to the work of health care providers, although it may be perceived as taboo by some. Providers can be advocates in a variety of ways, and those opportunities may vary over time or in one's professional versus citizen role. This could include working with health care leadership to improve connections between health care and CBOs or writing or speaking to the community about the importance of these connections. Blancato concurred and told health care providers and others with frontline experience—whether at the medical, hospital, or community level—that they are the most authentic advocates.

From Huang's perspective, the workshop presentations and discussions make it clear that a shift is coming in how people in medicine and policy circles think about the importance of nutrition and dietary assessment in public health. It is a purposeful shift for those who were trained in the medication-oriented model of addressing health, toward more opportunities and funding for educating providers about nutrition and providing nutrition services in the community. DiMaria-Ghalili added that training on social determinants of health is being integrated into health care provider curricula, which is a major shift but one that sets the stage for better equipping providers to address food and nutrition insecurity and malnutrition.

REFERENCES

Adams, K. M., K. C. Lindell, M. Kohlmeier, and S. H. Zeisel. 2006. Status of nutrition education in medical schools. *American Journal of Clinical Nutrition* 83(4):941S–944S.

Barker, L. A., B. S. Gout, and T. C. Crowe. 2011. Hospital malnutrition: Prevalence, identification and impact on patients and the healthcare system. *International Journal of Environmental Research and Public Health* 8(2):514–527.

Blancato, R., and M. Whitmire. 2021. The crucial role of federal nutrition programs in promoting health among low-income older adults. *Generations* 45(2):1–11.

Bradley, E. H., B. R. Elkins, J. Herrin, and B. Elbel. 2011. Health and social services expenditures: Associations with health outcomes. *BMJ Quality and Safety* 20(10):826–831.

Chin, M. H. 2020. Advancing health equity in patient safety: A reckoning, challenge and opportunity. *BMJ Quality and Safety.*

Chin, M. H. 2021. New horizons—addressing healthcare disparities in endocrine disease: Bias, science, and patient care. *International Journal of Clinical Endocrinology and Metabolism* 106(12):e4887–e4902.

Curriculum Committee of the Nutrition Academic Award Program. 2002. *Nutrition curriculum guide for training physicians.* https://www.nhlbi.nih.gov/sites/default/files/media/docs/NAA%20Nutrition%20Curriculum%20Guide.pdf (accessed September 14, 2022).

de Lorgeril, M., P. Salen, J. L. Martin, I. Monjaud, J. Delaye, and N. Mamelle. 1999. Mediterranean diet, traditional risk factors, and the rate of cardiovascular complications after myocardial infarction: Final report of the Lyon Diet Heart Study. *Circulation* 99(6):779–785.

Frank, E., J. Breyan, and L. Elon. 2000. Physician disclosure of healthy personal behaviors improves credibility and ability to motivate. *Archives of Family Medicine* 9(3):287–290.

GAO (United States Government Accountability Office). 2019. *Nutrition assistance programs: Agencies could do more to help address the nutritional needs of older adults.* GAO.

Gray, K.F. and Cunnyngham, K., 2016. Trends in supplemental nutrition assistance program participation rates: Fiscal year 2010 to fiscal year 2015 (No. 83167c08faee4195a-b0168e9f16dffd5). Mathematica Policy Research.

Kaye, N. 2021. *Massachusetts fosters partnerships between Medicaid accountable care and community organizations to improve health outcomes.* https://www.nashp.org/massachusetts-fosters-partnerships-between-medicaid-accountable-care-and-community-organizations-to-improve-health-outcomes (accessed August 8, 2022).

Kinderknecht, K., G. Rampersad, J. Romero, and T. Simmons. 2022. *Hunger health equity.* Health Equity Action League of Feeding America.

Kreuter, M. W., S. G. Chheda, and F. C. Bull. 2000. How does physician advice influence patient behavior? Evidence for a priming effect. *Archives of Family Medicine* 9(5):426–433.

Kushner, R. F., L. Van Horn, C. L. Rock, M. S. Edwards, C. W. Bales, M. Kohlmeier, and S. R. Akabas. 2014. Nutrition education in medical school: A time of opportunity. *The American Journal of Clinical Nutrition* 99(5):1167S–1173S.

Leong, B., D. Ren, D. Monlezun, D. Ly, L. Sarris, and T. S. Harlan. 2014. Teaching third and fourth year medical students how to cook: An innovative approach to training students in lifestyle modification for chronic disease management. *Medical Science Educator* 24(1):43.

Martinson, K., R. Koralek, E. Harbison, and L. Wherry. 2006. *Early implementation of the Minnesota Integrated Services Project.* Washington, DC: The Urban Institute

McConnell, K. J. 2016. Oregon's Medicaid coordinated care organizations. *JAMA* 315(9):869–870.

Mozaffarian, D., S. Y. Angell, T. Lang, and J. A. Rivera. 2018. Role of government policy in nutrition-barriers to and opportunities for healthier eating. *BMJ* 361:k2426.

Mozaffarian, D., S. Fleischhacker, and J. R. Andres. 2021. Prioritizing nutrition security in the U.S. *JAMA* 325(16):1605–1606.

NASEM (National Academies of Sciences, Engineering, and Medicine). 2020. *Social isolation and loneliness in older adults: Opportunities for the health care system.* Washington, DC: The National Academies Press.

National Research Council Committee on Nutrition in Medical Education. 1985. In *Nutrition education in U.S. medical schools.* Washington, DC: National Academies Press.

Nicklett, E. J., K. E. Johnson, L. M. Troy, M. Vartak, and A. Reiter. 2021. Food access, diet quality, and nutritional status of older adults during COVID-19: A scoping review. *Frontiers in Public Health* 9:763994.

Pang, B., Z. Memem, C. Diamant, E. Clarke, S. Chou, and H. Gregory. 2019. Culinary medicine and community partnership: Hands-on culinary skills training to empower medical students to provide patient-centered nutrition education. *Medical Education Online* 24(1):1630238.

Robert Wood Johnson Foundation. 2017. Visualizing health equity: One size does not fit all infographic. https://www.rwjf.org/en/library/infographics/visualizing-health-equity.html (accessed September 14, 2022).

Sacks, F. M., G. A. Bray, V. J. Carey, S. R. Smith, D. H. Ryan, S. D. Anton, K. McManus, C. M. Champagne, L. M. Bishop, N. Laranjo, M. S. Leboff, J. C. Rood, L. de Jonge, F. L. Greenway, C. M. Loria, E. Obarzanek, and D. A. Williamson. 2009. Comparison of weight-loss diets with different compositions of fat, protein, and carbohydrates. *New England Journal of Medicine* 360(9):859–873.

Smith, D. R. 2008. The historical decline of tobacco smoking among United States physicians: 1949–1984. *Tobacco Induced Diseases* 4:9.

Stauber, Z., A. C. Razavi, L. Sarris, T. S. Harlan, and D. J. Monlezun. 2022. Multisite medical student-led community culinary medicine classes improve patients' diets: Machine learning-augmented propensity score-adjusted fixed effects cohort analysis of 1381 subjects. *American Journal of Lifestyle Medicine* 16(2):214–220.

Trichopoulou, A., T. Costacou, C. Bamia, and D. Trichopoulos. 2003. Adherence to a Mediterranean diet and survival in a Greek population. *New England Journal of Medicine* 348(26):2599–2608.

Appendix A

Workshop Agendas

**Workshop 1: Dietary and Nutrition Assessments in
Older Adults: Foundations and Current Status**

April 8, 2022
1:00 PM–3:00 PM EDT

1:00 PM	**Introduction: Demographic Change** Heather Keller, Schlegel-UW Research Institute for Aging and University of Waterloo
1:10	**nutritionDAY** Dorothee Volkert, Friedrich-Alexander-University of Erlangen-Nürnberg
1:20	**Baltimore Longitudinal Study of Aging and the InCHIANTI Study** Luigi Ferrucci, National Institute on Aging, National Institutes of Health
1:30	**NHANES** Shinyoung Jun, Purdue University
1:40	**NHATS** Rose Ann DiMaria-Ghalili, College of Nursing and Health Professions, Drexel University

1:50	**Amsterdam Cohort** Marjolein Visser, Vrije Universiteit Amsterdam
2:00	**Panel Discussion with Speakers** Moderated by Heather Keller and Regan Bailey

**Workshop 2: Advances and Key Issues in
Dietary Assessments of Older Adults**

April 22, 2022
1:00 PM–3:00 PM EDT

1:00 PM	**Introduction: Assessing Nutrition Risk Among Community Dwelling Rural Older Adults: The Geisinger Rural Aging Study** Diane C. Mitchell, Pennsylvania State University
1:15	**Georgia Centenarian Study** Mary Ann Johnson, Department of Nutrition and Health Sciences at the University of Nebraska-Lincoln
1:35	**Adopting Diverse Dietary Assessment Methods Among Community Dwelling Adults or Clinical Nursing Home Residents** Jeanne de Vries, Wageningen, The Netherlands
1:55	**Assessing Dietary Intakes Among Adults from Diverse Populations** Katherine L. Tucker, University of Massachusetts Lowell
2:15	**Using Technological Approaches to Record Dietary Intakes Among Adults** Marie Kainoa Fialkowski Revilla, University of Hawai'i at Mānoa
2:35	**Panel Discussion with Speakers** Moderated by Carol Boushey and Diane Mitchell

Workshop 3: Nutritional Screening in Older Adults

April 29, 2022
1:00 PM–3:00 PM EDT

1:00 PM   **Introduction: Screening for Undernutrition in Older Adults from the U.S.: From the Nutrition Screening Initiative to 2022**
Gordon Jensen, University of Vermont

1:15   **Screening for Undernutrition in Older Adults: The International Experience**
Marian de van der Schueren, Han University

1:40   **Screening for Food Insecurity**
Heather Eicher-Miller, Purdue University

2:05   **Danish Experiences with Screening**
Sussi Friis Buhl, University of Southern Denmark

2:30   **Panel Discussion with Speakers**
Moderated by Gordon Jensen and Claire Corish

Workshop 4: Advances and Key Issues in Dietary Assessments of Older Adults

May 6, 2022
1:00 PM–3:00 PM EDT

1:00 PM   **Introduction**
Elbert Huang, University of Chicago

1:10   **Education Policy: Education of Health Professionals**
Timothy Harlan, George Washington University

1:30   **Food Policy: Meals on Wheels**
Ucheoma Akobundu, Meals on Wheels

1:50   **Health Care Payment Policy: Food Insecurity and Medicare Alternative Payment Models**
Marshall Chin, University of Chicago

2:10   **The Big Picture and New Legislation**
Bob Blancato, Defeat Malnutrition Today

2:30   **Panel Discussion with Speakers**
Moderated by Rose Ann DiMaria-Ghalili and Elbert Huang

Appendix B

Abbreviations and Acronyms

ACO   accountable care organization
AHEI   Alternate Healthy Eating Index
ASA24®   Automated Self-Administered 24-hour Dietary Assessment
           Tool

BLSA   Baltimore Longitudinal Study on Aging
BMI   body mass index

CBO   community-based organization

DHA   docosahexaenoic acid
DST   Dietary Screening Tool

FFQ   food frequency questionnaire

GLIM   Global Leadership Initiative in Malnutrition
GNRI   Geriatric Nutrition Risk Index
GRAS   Geisinger Rural Aging Study

MaNuEL   Malnutrition in the Elderly
MIND   Mediterranean-DASH intervention for Neurodegenerative
           Delay
MNA   Mini Nutritional Assessment®

| MST | Malnutrition Screening Tool |
| MUST | Malnutrition Universal Screening Tool |

NHANES	National Health and Nutrition Examination Survey
NHATS	National Health and Aging Trends Study
NIH	National Institutes of Health
NRI	Nutritional Risk Index
NRS	Nutritional Risk Screening
NRS-2002	Danish Nutritional Risk Screening-2002
NUFFE	Nutritional Form for the Elderly

| OAA | Older Americans Act |

SCREEN	Seniors in the Community: Risk Evaluation for Eating and Nutrition
SGA	Subjective Global Assessment
SNAP	Supplemental Nutrition Assistance Program
SNAQ	Short Nutritional Assessment Questionnaire

| UN | United Nations |

| WHO | World Health Organization |

Appendix C

Biographical Sketches of Planning Committee Members

Regan L. Bailey, Ph.D., M.P.H., R.D., is associate institute director for the Institute for Advancing Health through Agriculture and professor of nutrition at Texas A&M University. She previously served as a professor of nutrition science at Purdue University, and as a nutritional epidemiologist and director of career development at the National Institutes of Health, Office of Dietary Supplements. Dr. Bailey completed her dietetic internship and M.S. in Food and Nutrition from the Indiana University of Pennsylvania. Dr. Bailey received her Ph.D. in Nutrition Science from the Pennsylvania State University and her M.P.H from the Bloomberg School of Public Health at Johns Hopkins University. Her research focuses on improving the methods of measuring nutritional status to optimize health. She utilizes nationally representative survey data to characterize the American dietary landscape, to identify the optimal methods for assessment of biomarkers of nutritional status, and to understand how dietary intakes relate to health outcomes. Dr. Bailey worked to develop the first models combining nutrients from foods and dietary supplements to estimate total usual intake. Her work was used to inform the calcium and vitamin D Dietary Reference Intakes and the National Academy reference values. Dr. Bailey has used these models to identify differences in nutritional exposures by gender, race, ethnicity, life stage, and income, suggesting the need for population-specific interventions and policy. She has authored more than 150 peer-reviewed scientific publications. Dr. Bailey served on the 2020 Dietary Guidelines for American Advisory Committee, and as chair of the Data Analysis and Food

Pattern Modeling Subcommittee. She was a member of National Academy of Medicine's 2021 Committee on Scanning for New Evidence on Riboflavin to Support a Dietary Reference Intake Review.

Carol J. Boushey, Ph.D., M.P.H., is associate research professor, Epidemiology Program, at the University of Hawai'i Cancer Center and holds an adjunct professor position in the Nutrition Science Department, Purdue University. She specializes in evaluating dietary exposures with an emphasis on technology, diverse racial/ethnic groups, and dietary patterns associated with health or risk for disease. Dr. Boushey is involved with the dietary assessment methods used with the Multiethnic Cohort representing five ethnic groups (Japanese American, Hawaiian, non-Hispanic White, African American, Hispanic/Latino). She has participated in two National Academies committee reports addressing the process used to establish and optimize the Dietary Guidelines for Americans. Dr. Boushey was appointed to the 2020 Dietary Guidelines Advisory Committee and assumed the Chair of the Dietary Patterns Subcommittee. She focused on foods and nutrition for her undergraduate degree at the University of Washington (UW) which included a semester at the University of Copenhagen, Denmark. Her dietetic internship combined with a Masters of Public Health included medical rotations in Hawaii and a Public Health rotation with the Louisiana Department of Health. Her Ph.D. degree from UW focused on dietary intake and risk for disease through the interdisciplinary nutrition program and the epidemiology program.

Clare Corish, Ph.D., is a professor of clinical nutrition & dietetics and the programme director for the MSc in Clinical Nutrition & Dietetics at the School of Public Health, Physiotherapy and Sports Science, at the University College Dublin. She is a CORU registered dietitian and has a long-standing commitment to nutrition research activities, particularly in disease-related malnutrition and malnutrition in the older person. Dr. Corish is an active member of the Irish Nutrition & Dietetic Institute (INDI) and the Nutrition Society holding several leadership roles in the past including INDI president and chair of the Nutrition Society Irish Section. She was a member of the Food Safety Authority of Ireland Public Health Nutrition subcommittee from 2012–2021 and has served on a number of expert committees over many years. Dr. Corish is a member of the Editorial board of the U.S. *Journal of the Academy of Nutrition and Dietetics,* the U.S. Association for Nutrition journal, *Nutrition Today,* and the Australian journal *Nutrition and Dietetics* as well as being a peer reviewer for many high impact nutrition journals.

Rose Ann DiMaria-Ghalili, Ph.D., R.N., FASPEN, FAAN, FGSA, is the associate dean for interprofessional research and development and a professor of nursing in the College of Nursing and Health Professions (CNHP), with courtesy appointments in the nutrition science department and School of Biomedical Engineering at Drexel University. She is a geriatric nurse scientist and her research focuses on integrating nutrition and novel technologies to improve health outcomes and quality of life for older adults with acute and chronic conditions across the care continuum. Recognizing the need to improve the measurement of nutritional intake, Dr. DiMaria-Ghalili led a team of engineers on the research and development of a patented wireless device to track and monitor fluid intake. Dr. DiMaria-Ghalili serves as the principal investigator of the Cell2Society Aging Research Network (Cell-2Society), a Drexel Area of Research Excellence (DARE) initiative, where she leads a team working to create a novel ecosystem for the pursuit of use-inspired aging research. Dr. DeMaria-Ghalili is a Distinguished Educator in Gerontological Nursing, a recognition from the National Hartford Center for Gerontological Nursing Excellence. She is a fellow in the American Society for Parenteral and Enteral Nutrition (ASPEN), and a recipient of the ASPEN's Dudrick Research Scholar Award and of the ASPEN's Distinguished Nutrition Support Nurse Service Award. Dr. DiMaria-Ghalili has previously presented on nutrition during care transitions at a National Academies workshop.

Elbert S. Huang, M.D., M.P.H., is professor of medicine and public health sciences and director of the Center for Chronic Disease Research and Policy at the University of Chicago. Dr. Huang is an international leader in the study of diabetes in older people. Older people are a highly heterogeneous group, with the sickest frequently excluded from clinical trials. Using techniques from health economics, simulation modeling, and analysis of real-world data, Dr. Huang has characterized the heterogeneity of the older diabetes population, the modern natural history of disease, and illustrated the impact of patient health status on the benefits of glycemic control. This research has directly influenced care guidelines that now emphasize (1) individualization of glycemic goals by health status, (2) the role of patient treatment preferences, (3) the clinical importance of hypoglycemia, and (4) management of geriatric conditions. Dr. Huang is an elected member of the American Society for Clinical Investigation. He received his A.B., M.D., and M.P.H. from Harvard and came to the University of Chicago in 2001. Dr. Huang has previously served as a panelist for the National Academy meeting on Multiple Chronic Conditions and Clinical Guidelines.

Gordon L. Jensen, M.D., Ph.D., became senior associate dean for research and professor of medicine and nutrition at the Larner College of Medicine, University of Vermont in 2016. From 2007–2015 he served as professor and head of nutritional sciences at Penn State University and professor of medicine at the Penn State College of Medicine. He was at Vanderbilt University Medical Center from 1998–2007 where he was director of the Vanderbilt Center for Human Nutrition and professor of medicine. He received his M.D. from Cornell University Medical College and his Ph.D. in nutritional biochemistry from Cornell University. He completed residency training in Internal Medicine and fellowship training in Clinical Nutrition at New England Deaconess Hospital, Harvard Medical School. He is a past president of the American Society for Nutrition (ASN), a past president of the American Society for Parenteral and Enteral Nutrition (ASPEN), and a past chair of the Association of Nutrition Programs and Departments. He served two terms as a member of the Food and Nutrition Board. His research interests have focused on the impact of nutritional status on health and functional outcomes in older persons. He has authored more than 205 journal articles, reviews, and book chapters.

Heather H. Keller, Ph.D., R.D., FDC FCAHS, is the Schlegel Research Chair in Nutrition & Aging at Schlegel-UW Research Institute for Aging and a professor at the University of Waterloo. She is an internationally recognized expert in geriatric nutrition, assessment, and treatment. Research areas focus on nutrition risk and malnutrition identification and treatment across care sectors; improving nutrition care processes and implementing screening and other best practices; supporting food intake of diverse groups living in the community, including those living with dementia; and improving hospital and residential food and promoting food intake and the mealtime experience in these settings. Dr. Keller is a founding member and past chair/co-chair (2009–2018) of the Canadian Malnutrition Task Force. She was accepted into the Canadian Academy of Health Sciences in 2018 and is a Fellow of Dietitians of Canada. Dr. Keller trained at Western University (Ph.D., Epidemiology & Biostatistics), McGill University (MSc Human Nutrition) and University of Guelph (BASc, Human Nutrition).

Diana C. Mitchell, M.S., R.D., received her graduate degree in nutrition from The Pennsylvania State University and is a registered dietitian with membership in the Academy for Nutrition and Dietetics and the American Society for Nutrition. She currently serves as an associate research professor and the director of the Diet Assessment Center in the Department of Nutritional Sciences at The Pennsylvania State University where she has been for more than 30 years. In this role she is responsible for managing all external and internal research studies with dietary outcomes, including funding acquisition, proposal development, budget administration, and manuscript development. Her research interests include developing, validating, and improving various diet assessment methodologies, dietary patterns, diet quality, and population-based dietary exposure research. For more than 22 years, she has coordinated the diet assessment for the Geisinger Rural Aging Study, a longitudinal study of 20,000 older adults residing in Pennsylvania. This project has provided the expertise in developing and refining methodology to assess diets in older adults that has led to over 30 publications highlighting dietary intake methodology, diet quality, and diet as it relates to other health outcomes.